Literary Lives

General Editor: **Richard Dutton**, Professor of English, Lancaster University

This series offers stimulating accounts of the literary careers of the most admired and influential English-language authors. Volumes follow the outline of the writers' working lives, not in the spirit of traditional biography, but aiming to trace the professional, publishing and social contexts which shaped their writing.

Published titles include:

Clinton Machann
MATTHEW ARNOLD

Jan Fergus
JANE AUSTEN

Tom Winnifrith and Edward Chitham
CHARLOTTE AND EMILY BRONTË

Sarah Wood
ROBERT BROWNING

Janice Farrar Thaddeus
FRANCES BURNEY

Caroline Franklin
BYRON

Nancy A. Walker
KATE CHOPIN

Roger Sales
JOHN CLARE

Cedric Watts
JOSEPH CONRAD

Grahame Smith
CHARLES DICKENS

George Parfitt
JOHN DONNE

Paul Hammond
JOHN DRYDEN

Kerry McSweeney
GEORGE ELIOT

Tony Sharpe
T. S. ELIOT

Harold Pagliaro
HENRY FIELDING

Mary Lago
E. M. FORSTER

James Gibson
THOMAS HARDY

Gerald Roberts
GERARD MANLEY HOPKINS

Kenneth Graham
HENRY JAMES

W. David Kaye
BEN JONSON

John Worthen
D. H. LAWRENCE

Angela Smith
KATHERINE MANSFIELD

Lisa Hopkins
CHRISTOPHER MARLOWE

Cedric C. Brown
JOHN MILTON

Peter Davison
GEORGE ORWELL

Linda Wagner-Martin
SYLVIA PLATH

Felicity Rosslyn
ALEXANDER POPE

Richard Dutton
WILLIAM SHAKESPEARE

John Williams
MARY SHELLEY

Michael O'Neill
PERCY BYSSHE SHELLEY

Gary Waller
EDMUND SPENSER

Tony Sharpe
WALLACE STEVENS

Joseph McMinn
JONATHAN SWIFT

Leonée Ormond
ALFRED TENNYSON

Peter Shillingsburg
WILLIAM MAKEPEACE THACKERAY

David Wykes
EVELYN WAUGH

John Mepham
VIRGINIA WOOLF

John Williams
WILLIAM WORDSWORTH

Alasdair D. F. Macrae
W. B. YEATS

Literary Lives
Series Standing Order ISBN 0–333–71486–5 hardcover
Series Standing Order ISBN 0–333–80334–5 paperback
(outside North America only)

You can receive future titles in this series as they are published by placing a standing order. Please contact your bookseller or, in case of difficulty, write to us at the address below with your name and address, the title of the series and one of the ISBNs quoted above.

Customer Services Department, Macmillan Distribution Ltd, Houndmills, Basingstoke, Hampshire RG21 6XS, England

John Clare

A Literary Life

Roger Sales
Professor of English
School of English and American Studies
University of East Anglia

palgrave

First published 2002 by
PALGRAVE
Houndmills, Basingstoke, Hampshire RG21 6XS and
175 Fifth Avenue, New York, N. Y. 10010
Companies and representatives throughout the world

PALGRAVE is the new global academic imprint of St. Martin's Press LLC Scholarly and Reference Division and Palgrave Publishers Ltd (formerly Macmillan Press Ltd).

ISBN 0–333–65270–3 hardback
ISBN 0–333–65271–1 paperback

This book is printed on paper suitable for recycling and made from fully managed and sustained forest sources.

Cataloguing-in-publication data

A catalogue record for this book is available from the British Library.

A catalogue record for this book is available from the Library of Congress.

10 9 8 7 6 5 4 3 2 1
11 10 09 08 07 06 05 04 03 02

Printed and bound in Great Britain by
Antony Rowe Ltd, Chippenham, Wiltshire

Good Angels be my Guard:
For Sarah and Adrian

Contents

Acknowledgements

I am grateful once again to Janet Todd, herself the author of a book on Clare, for her encouragement and example as far as my own writing of literary and cultural history is concerned. The pleasure of writing this book has been mixed with great sadness at the untimely death of Roger Pipe-Fowler, a close friend and an exemplary colleague who gave me (and many others) so much good advice over the years. Past colleagues who have influenced my work on literature and history include David Aers, Ros Ballaster, Sarah Beckwith, David Lawton, George MacLennan (who has written well on Clare and madness) and Philip O'Neill. For this book I am also grateful to Roger Cooter and Tim Marshall, who gave me some valuable help with medical histories, and to Robert Clark for discussions of the literary history of the Regency period.

A number of those in what is becoming known as the Clare community have helped me in matters great and small and I am very grateful to them. I acknowledge individual debts to them and others in some of the endnotes. It will be seen there that some Clare scholars are generous almost to a fault in sharing the fruits of their own labours. Jan Fergus's volume on Jane Austen in this series has been a model and very often an inspiration. Other Austen specialists who have helped me to understand this period better include Claudia L. Johnson and Anne K. Mellor. Editors who have recently asked me write on the Regency and early Victorian periods include Kate Campbell, Deidre Lynch, Judy Simons and Frances Wilson. Journals such as *Albion* and *Literature and History* have also kept me up to scratch with requests for reviews of books about the Regency period.

The endnotes give details of the archives that I have visited and I need to thank all those who have helped me with this material. In addition to the Clare collections at Northampton and Peterborough as well as archives in London, I have worked in libraries at Aberdeen, Chelmsford, Lincoln, Manchester, Matlock, Sheffield, Stamford and York. The rest of the research was done in the University Library at Cambridge which, as always, provided an extremely supportive environment. I just wish, as Clare once said about London, that we could creep a little closer to each other. Perhaps we shall, although I suspect that I shall have to do all of the creeping. Alex Noel-Tod, the subject specialist librarian at East Anglia, has also been a help. I would like to thank my publishers and various editors (Charmian Hearne and Eleanor Birne) for being very patient, and my university for a period of study leave during which the book was completed. My department kindly provided some extra funds for travel expenses. A number of people were kind enough to help me with my career when I had just started working on this book: Isobel Armstrong, Elizabeth Bronfen, Richard Dutton, Elizabeth Esteve-Coll, Kelvin Everest, Louis James, David Punter, Michael Robinson and Lorna Sage. I am grateful to them (and feel a tremendous sense of both personal and professional loss after Lorna's death earlier in the year). I am additionally much indebted to Richard Dutton who, as editor of this series, has been extremely prompt in offering sound comments and advice. An important and influential part of my career has been spent teaching in Germany. In addition to Elizabeth Bronfen, I would like to thank yet again Elfi Bettinger, Irmgard Maassen and Werner von Koppenfels for their encouragement and support. It should go without saying, but never quite does, that while I have received much help with this book I alone remain responsible for its content.

With a bit of help from Mr Rochester, this book is dedicated with love to all my good angels, particularly my sister Sarah and her family. My mother, from whose house back in Yorkshire I was able to visit a lot of the archives, helped me in so many different ways, not least because she is herself one of the very best historians that I know. I also read most of my microfilmed material while back there and would like to thank the members of the staff of the Doncaster Public Library for their help. I hope that my children, Will and Jess, will enjoy the book and appreciate why I felt it was important to spend a number of years thinking and writing about Clare. I am also grateful to Anne. I realised it was probably time to finish off the book when I went a few rounds late one night with a Regency boxer known as the Game Chicken, who makes a brief appearance in the last chapter. It was a scary experience. More seriously, I freely admit to having been disturbed at times when doing some of the archive work on madness that appears in the second part of the book and some readers may feel the same. It took me to places and mental spaces that I sometimes wished I was not visiting. It was however necessary to cover this area in archival depth since, with important exceptions that are referenced in the argument itself, it was one of the gaps in Clare criticism. Roy Porter's work was very influential here, and I am particularly grateful to him, as will become clear later.

I do not teach Clare on a regular basis, although the students over the years who have taken my Nineteenth Century Underworld course will recognise some of the material discussed here. I am grateful to all of them for making this course one of the high points in my teaching career. I have always done a lot of team-teaching, which I enjoy, and would like to thank my current partners: Kit Carver, Lynda Thompson and Kate Webb. Graduate students and others with whom I have discussed this book include Antje Blank, Graham Caveney, Victoria Christie, Glen Creeber, Kate Drayton, Karen Harris, Penny Hender, Bill Hughes, Mia Madey and Himansu Mohapatra. I am also grateful to Allan Lloyd-Smith. Perhaps this crazy gang can all meet at the Poets and Peasants Café Bar in Norwich when the book is published.

Textual Note and Chronology

The following abbreviations have been used to make it easier to supply in-text references and shorter endnotes:

AW *John Clare's Autobiographical Writings* (Oxford: Oxford University Press, 1986), Eric Robinson (ed.)

B *Byron* (Oxford: Oxford University Press, 1986), Jerome J. McGann (ed.)

BH *John Clare By Himself* (Manchester: Carcanet, 1996), Eric Robinson and David Powell (eds.)

CH *Clare: The Critical Heritage* (London: Routledge & Kegan Paul, 1973), Mark Storey (ed.)

EG Egerton Manuscripts, Letters Addressed to John Clare, British Library, 6 vols, 2245–50

EP *The Early Poems of John Clare 1804–1822* (Oxford: Clarendon Press, 1989), 2 vols, Eric Robinson and David Powell (eds.)

LJC *The Letters of John Clare* (Oxford: Clarendon Press, 1985), Mark Storey (ed.)

LP *The Later Poems of John Clare 1837–1864* (Oxford: Clarendon Press, 1984), 2 vols, Eric Robinson and David Powell (eds.)

MP *John Clare Poems of the Middle Period 1822–1837* (Oxford: Clarendon Press, 1996), 2 vols, Eric Robinson et al. (eds.)

All quotations throughout abide by what I and my publishers understand to be the accepted guidelines for fair dealing in respect of research and criticism. Most quotations from nineteenth-century newspapers and periodicals are provided with in-text references. The endnotes are primarily concerned to identify the sources for quotations: full publication details are given on first citation and thereafter abbreviations are used. There are, however, some fuller, more descriptive notes particularly in relation to social and cultural history. The notes to the last chapter, which deals with Byron, also tend towards the full and descriptive simply because so much has been written about him. As will become clear, I am mainly concerned to identify the particular nature of Clare's ambiguous relationship with him. I found, however, that in order to do this there had to be some more free-standing work on Byron and the Byronic. I have also more occasionally thought it appropriate to show other Clare specialists which sources I am using, even though a book like this is obviously not intended to be a scholarly monograph aimed primarily at them but, rather, at students and general readers. I very much hope nevertheless that, as they have worked in some of the same archives as me, I have managed to give them a reasonably good sense of the research base for some of my arguments within the confines of a book like this. My third and fourth chapters on the early Victorian period introduce some archive material that may not be so familiar to Clare specialists.

This is my third book on Regency England, the others being *English Literature in History 1780–1830: Pastoral and Politics* (1983) and *Jane Austen and Representations of Regency England* (1994/6). The first of these includes a chapter on Clare which relates his versions of pastoral to those by writers such as William Cobbett, George Crabbe and William Wordsworth. It helped to establish an agenda about Clare's politics. I did not want, however, to repeat these arguments and was drawn back to writing about Clare in order to develop some different ones. First, and probably foremost, I wanted to suggest that the six volumes of letters addressed to Clare, when cross-referenced with his own letters, are one of the major, central sources for the literary history of this period. This has not been fully recognised because Clare still has a reputation as being a marginal figure. Mark Storey has published some of these letters addressed to Clare in editions listed above. There is still a need for an edition of them. It would be of great value to all students of this period, even if they are not particularly interested in Clare himself. I quote as much as possible in a book of this length from these letters to try to establish their importance.

My second main objective was to suggest that the term Regency needs to have a wider currency in Clare studies. Technically, this was the period from 1811 to 1820. I have nevertheless adopted a broader definition which sees the period as running from the 1790s through to the 1820s. I relate Clare's work and its reception to the Regency period, and then to the cultural shifts that took place as it was replaced by early Victorian mentalities. Clare has not been well served, as James McKusick and others have noticed, by literary histories that privilege Romanticism as the key term, particularly Wordsworthian or visionary Romanticism. Conventional definitions of Romanticism have also, as Anne K. Mellor and others have pointed out, helped to marginalise important writings by women. I do not want to claim for a moment that seeing Clare as a Regency writer solves all the problems about contextualising his work. I am strongly of the view, however, that the term Regency is extremely useful in foregrounding his relationship with the

London Magazine. I have taken this to be a crucial part of his literary life, suggesting that even the asylum writings and performances are still dominated by the Regency agendas of this magazine. I suggest more particularly that John Scott, the first editor of the *London* who had also worked as a journalist in Stamford, needs to be seen as a significant influence on Clare's literary life.

A third objective was to place Clare's literary life in contexts provided by other working-class writers. Clare was an agricultural labourer, who eventually achieved some recognition as a published poet. Although I am in part following up important work done here by John Goodridge and others, my sense has always been that there are still some critics who feel that Clare's achievements are always in danger of being devalued if there is too much discussion of minor and forgotten writers. His reputation is thought to be best served by relating his work to that of, say, Byron rather than to that of, say, Robert Bloomfield. My argument throughout is that it is important to do both. I do not think that it is possible to understand Clare's literary life without looking in some detail at the way in which other peasant-poets and artisan-poets, as well as working-class Regency boxers, were constructed and marketed. The point requires emphasis since, unless it is accepted, it might seem at times that Clare is disappearing from this narrative of his literary life. Yet the stories of these other figures are an important and indeed vital way of understanding his own.

I have already indicated that a fourth starting point was the feeling that there was more to be said about asylum culture and Clare's place within it. I reject quite emphatically the view that he was indeed mad during the early asylum years and wonder just how sane the mad-doctors might have been. If he did eventually go mad, then this was something that was probably produced by asylum culture itself. Just as I tell the stories of other working-class figures in order to illuminate Clare's literary life, so I try to recover the lives of others who were deemed to be mad. This is once again not to displace Clare himself from the narrative but, on the contrary, to suggest that his experiences and writings need to be read alongside other life stories. The fact that he may not himself have known these stories is not at all relevant to the way in which the argument proceeds.

I am using editions that reproduce Clare's writings with his own spellings, known as the Clarendon editions. This book would not have been possible without these editions. When I first started working on Clare, it was necessary to do a lot of raw archive work before important literary and historical questions could even be posed. This is no longer the case. Readers may initially experience some difficulty with some quotations, but after a bit will get used to them, particularly if, as John Lucas puts it, they read with the ear as well as with the eye. The editions in question are still expensive ones to be consulted in libraries by most students. There are, however, a number of good selected editions available for those who may just be embarking on a study of Clare, such as Kelsey Thornton's one in the Everyman Poets series and John Goodridge's one in the Wordsworth Poetry Library. There is a more substantial paperback edition, complete with scholarly notes, by Eric Robinson and David Powell in the Oxford Authors series. This is the one recommended for students who are doing detailed research on Clare.

It has not been possible in a book of this length to deal with all aspects of this long literary life. I say relatively little about the way in which Clare was edited during his lifetime as I regard this, and some of the partisan responses that it provokes, as a bit of a blind alley. I nevertheless say enough at the end of the second chapter to give readers a general sense of the arguments. I am a literary and cultural historian rather than an editor, and felt that I could employ myself more usefully elsewhere. Although I reference studies of Clare's indebtedness to the folk tradition, I concentrate on his relationships with more mainstream literary culture (for instance, my work on the *London Magazine* and Byron). Here I am following the lead of a number of younger Clare scholars, who have made me realise just how literary Clare was in a perhaps old-fashioned sense of the term. I had underestimated this in my earlier work. This is not to deny the importance of the folk tradition, and readers who are primarily interested in this aspect of Clare's literary life should consult the detailed and scholarly notes in the Clarendon editions as well as important studies by George Deacon and others, which as indicated are referenced in my argument. Very much prompted by others, however, I just felt that it was time to tell a different story.

Lucas refers, as will be seen, to Clare's great literary expectations, pointing forward to Charles Dickens's novel. Although a book like this one needs to cover as much of the waterfront as possible, it also makes sense to spend longer at some places on it than at others. My story about Clare's literary life is one about the way in which he was driven by these great literary expectations which, given the class system then, there was never any real hope of him fulfilling. He was first marketed in 1820 as a Northamptonshire Peasant and could never shake off this label or brandname despite the quality and quantity of his work: that is the literary life in a nutshell. He was not able to join the literary profession except in this very tokenistic, condescending way.

This may, at first glance, seem to be a bleak and depressing story. I argue nevertheless, explicitly right at the end of the book and more implicitly throughout, that the opposite may be the case. I see Clare as a great survivor and suggest that this is why he has become such a writer's writer (something which is documented in the endnotes). He wrote because he had to write: as simple and as complicated as that. There was a relatively brief period in the early 1820s when his writing reached an audience. There were also longer periods, when he first started writing and then again during his imprisonment in lunatic asylums from 1837 to 1864, when almost nobody seemed to be listening. He just carried on writing, no matter whether there were readers or not. This is not, then, a depressing literary life but rather in many ways an uplifting one. It is about the pleasures, or to use one of Clare's keywords, the joy of writing. He uses the words joy or joys more than ten times in a relatively short poem entitled 'The Progress of Rhyme'. The asylum poetry often tried to recover the pleasure of writing. The words joy and joys occur over forty times in a relatively long poem such as 'Child Harold'. Although it would be easy enough to represent Clare as being a victim of snobbery and prejudice, I have chosen instead as indicated to see him as a survivor. He is also a survivor in the sense that, thanks to the diligence of his editors and others, his writings are more widely known and appreciated now than those of many nineteenth-century literary professionals. My book is about a survivor, as well as being itself a part of this process of literary survival.

Clare was an extremely prolific writer, as the Clarendon editions demonstrate. It has not been possible here to offer detailed readings of the full range of his work. The openness of some of his texts also often makes providing short quotations difficult. A literary life needs to combine readings with biographical details, and yet it is primarily an exercise in literary history rather than being a work of criticism or biography. As Jonathan Bate will shortly be publishing a major new biography of Clare, it was important to try to get the balance right so that these two books could complement rather than overlap too much with each other. I have therefore tried to place Clare in the literary history of the Regency and earlier Victorians periods, relating this as much as possible to a wider social and cultural history. I have conducted biographical research, largely through the six volumes of letters addressed to him, but this is still not a biography. I offer readings of some of his poetry and prose, while remaining aware of how much more could have been said about them. This is a literary life that is primarily concerned with constructions of literary and social identities, the marketing and transmission of them and the reception of them. As it is about these things, it was necessary to tell other life stories in order to illuminate Clare's own one. I emphasise, and perhaps labour, this point since it is crucial to an understanding of what this book tries to achieve, and what it does not try to achieve.

As Clare's literary life may not be familiar to many readers, I follow this textual note with a very brief chronology. There is a fuller one, produced by John Goodridge, on the Clare web-site which is referenced in the Further Reading section at the end of the book. Mark Storey's edition of the letters also contains a chronology.

1793	Born at Helpston on 13 July
c. 1803	Meets Mary Joyce while at school in Glinton. Had previously had some schooling in Helpston.
c. 1805	Begins work as a ploughboy. Starts writing poetry
1806	Buys James Thomson's *Seasons*
1807	Becomes a gardener at Burghley House
1812	Joins the Militia
1814	Meets a local bookseller called Henson
1817	Works as a lime-burner at Bridge Casterton
1818	Meets Edward Drury, a cousin of the London publisher John Taylor
1819	Meets Taylor
1820	Publication of *Poems Descriptive of Rural Life and Scenery*, priced at five shillings and sixpence, which goes into four editions; first trip to London; meets local aristocrats and gentry; marries Patty
1821	John Scott killed in duel; Taylor takes over the *London Magazine*; publication of *The Village Minstrel*
1822	Second visit to London
1823	Deaths of Robert Bloomfield and Octavius Gilchrist
1824	Third visit to London
1825	Death of his patron, Admiral Lord Radstock
1827	Publication of *The Shepherd's Calendar* after long delay
1828	Fourth visit to London; visit to Boston, Lincolnshire
1832	Moves to Northborough
1835	Publication of *The Rural Muse*
1837	Admitted to High Beach Asylum
1841	Writes 'Child Harold' and 'Don Juan'. Walks from High Beach almost all the way home; admitted to Northampton General Lunatic Asylum
1850	William Knight, who transcribed many of his poems, leaves Northampton for another appointment
1864	Death
1865	Publication of Martin's biography

1
A Cage Glass All Round: Dilettante Patrons and Literary Philanthropists

Mistaken identities

As far as the reading public was concerned, Clare's literary life began very early in 1820 with the publication in London of *Poems Descriptive of Rural Life and Scenery, by John Clare, a Northamptonshire Peasant.* This volume, published by the progressive firm of Taylor and Hessey, which was already associated with John Keats's poetry, was widely reviewed and eventually went into four editions. Clare went to London for about a week, meeting his publisher John Taylor and some of those such as Admiral Lord Radstock and Eliza Emmerson who appointed themselves as his patrons. He also met some of the literary celebrities attached to the camp, bohemian *London Magazine*. Ironically enough, this Northamptonshire Peasant was by adoption a Cockney: Cockney Clare. He was to join Thomas De Quincey, William Hazlitt and Charles Lamb as a regular contributor to the *London*. He visited poets' corner at Westminster Abbey during this first visit to London. Would he ever be remembered there? The answer is not until 1989, which provides a snapshot of his literary life and its perceived marginality. Lord Byron got there first, as he usually did in Clare's experience, but only just, this particular time not being commemorated until the 1960s.

At home in Helpston, a straggling village (his own description) between Peterborough and Stamford, Clare found himself besieged with visitors. He had been born there in 1793, the year that the Revolutionary wars with France and her allies had begun. Although in his earlier life work sometimes took him away from this village for a time, he lived there until 1832 and then only moved a few miles down the road. He loved it and hated it. The carriages of the chattering classes beat a path to his door. Everybody seemed to want a slice of this literary action. Regency dandies and philanthropists were joined by both failed and aspiring writers hoping that some of Clare's rough literary magic would rub off on them. He became a 'strangers poppet Show' (*LJC*, p. 89) and a 'peep show' (*LJC*, p. 215). Some spectators were more interested in his sex life than his poetry: literary tourism shaded into a form of Regency sex tourism. He was also press-ganged into visiting the great and good in the locality, despite trying to continue to earn a living as an agricultural labourer. His local patrons were not used to taking no, or even maybe, for an answer from a Northamptonshire Peasant. Their wishes became his command. A clerical magistrate called Hopkinson sent a horse over to Helpston so that he did not have an excuse for not visiting: 'leaving me no option wether I chused to go or not' (*AW*, p. 121), even though it was harvest-time. Years later when another clergyman sent a horse for him he confessed that he was 'a bad horseman' (*LJC*, p. 432). Like most labourers, he was used to walking long distances. He postponed a visit to Burghley House, the seat of a local Tory grandee, the Marquis of Exeter, because of bad weather, fearing the embarrassment of arriving in dirty shoes. He had once worked in the gardens there, which had not proved to be a happy experience given a tyrannical head gardener and the fact that there was nothing to do but drink when work was over. One of the upper servants, sounding more aristo than the aristocracy despite the use of dialect, was mortified by this damned impudence and downright impertinence when Clare eventually arrived: 'you shoud stand for no weathers tho it rained knives and forks with the tynes (prongs) downward' (*AW*, p. 116). The Marquis himself was not nearly so put out as this haughty retainer, agreeing to pay Clare fifteen guineas a year.

Clare was also late in paying a visit to General Thomas Birch Reynardson at Holywell Hall, outside Stamford. The General bought his books in Stamford at a shop that had been taken over in 1818 by Edward Drury, who claimed the credit for discovering Clare as a writer. Drury had been on the knocker, actually visiting some of the big houses in the area to tell potential patrons about Clare.[1] Drury, who always had both eyes on the main chance, was hoping for great things from this connection with the Reynardsons. He told the publisher John Taylor, who was his cousin, that the General had plans for Clare to come to live and work at Holywell. The poet could have 'white bread or brown at the generals', the former being considered at this time as a luxury.[2]

The General and the poet appear to have met sometime in late January or early February at Drury's shop, where one of the items for sale was Clare himself as well as his poetry. Clare, having been scolded for not accepting an earlier invitation, eventually took the day off work and walked over to Holywell. He chose a fine spring day when it was not raining knives and forks with the prongs downwards. Drury sometimes acted as a fashion consultant for such visits. He sent the poet one of his own shirts in February for another visit to a big house, suggesting that it should be co-ordinated with a 'clean waistcoat' and 'nice silk handkerchief'.[3] Later on, Taylor gave Clare a smart black waistcoat and a 'dandyish' (*LJC*, p. 208) coat.

The General took Clare straightaway to admire the library, which was 'the largest I had seen then' (*AW*, p. 124). According to his own account, the poet was nevertheless not completely overawed by this setting or theatrical set. When the General proudly produced with a flourish a volume of elegies written by his father, the poet apparently spotted that they were imitations of James Hammond's *Love Elegies Written in the Year 1732*. Hammond's work had a preface by Lord Chesterfield and his life was eventually written by Dr Johnson: both pillars of polite eighteenth-century culture. Although it is not clear whether Clare actually voiced his opinions or not, the General's theatrical script for the patronage of a peasant-poet was not going entirely according to plan. This peasant-poet was better read in polite culture than he had any right, or reason, to be.

The General was so very proud of his library that he commissioned a catalogue of it in 1843 by a toady who sounds uncommonly like Austen's Mr Collins. Clare's first volume is the only one listed. This toady, in addition to waxing lyrical over the books and their setting, also praises some of the pictures. There was a Reubens and a Rembrandt, which no real gentry home should be without. Clare is, perhaps sullenly, silent about these treasures.[4] He made friends with a number of native painters later on and was 'fond of every thing relating to pictures' (*LJC*, p. 514).

The scene then shifts to the gardens, which the General was in the process of landscaping: 'a little river ran sweeping along and in one place he was forming a connection with it to form an Island' (*AW*, p. 125). Perhaps the plan was for Clare to work in these gardens and write a bit in his spare time, maybe in a picturesque little grotto, or hermitage.[5] The poet's eye is caught by a 'bird house built in the form of a cage glass all round and full of canarys that were fluttering about busily employd in building their nests –' (*AW*, p. 125). Clare does not mention explicitly the General's plans for him to live at Holywell as the family's very own tame pet poet and yet, in the image of the glass birdcage, comments on what such an experience might have been like. Once again, the General's script is coming unstuck. This poet has read far too much and may also be too independent to put up with the confinements of patronage.

Another character now enters the drama while Clare is strolling around the gardens. He thinks, first of all, that she must be the General's lady, only to discover that she is in fact the governess. He feels a fool for mistaking her identity, and yet the play is rapidly turning into one of mistaken identities. The General identifies himself to Drury as a benevolent patron, but in the event does next to nothing for Clare. He exits from the play just as quickly as he had entered it: he does not buy another volume of Clare's poetry. So much for supporting your local poet. He is perhaps warned off by a lack of deference in the poet's manner and manners. He identifies Clare as somebody who should have been ever so forelock-tugging grateful to drop absolutely everything for the rare and wonderful privilege of visiting Holywell, when such a visit might in fact have been very inconvenient. The poet is not completely overawed in the library and walks about the garden thinking about the restrictions of patronage. The governess dresses like a great lady but is not one. It is all very confusing. Identities are fluid. Characters are not who they seem to be. First impressions are dangerously deceptive.

Clare is bundled off to the servants' hall for his dinner, as was usually the case when he visited the big houses in his neighbourhood. It is not known whether he had white bread or brown, or both. Like the governess, he inhabits an awkward social space. He can be part of the family for a short time, even though he also has to be made acutely aware that he is apart from it. He meets the governess again after dinner and she suggests that they must write to each other. Once again, Clare is not being given much say in the matter. A governess's identity was bound up with setting standards of decorum and propriety for the children in her care. She controls the sexuality of others by governing her own. Yet she could also desire and be desired: Jane Eyre eventually marries Mr Rochester after the madwoman in the attic has destroyed herself, and perhaps also in a sense him as well, in Charlotte Brontë's novel. The legend is that Charlotte's brother, Branwell, had an affair with rich Mrs Robinson while acting as private tutor to one of her children. According to Clare's account, this governess is all but throwing herself at him. She affects to be interested in his newly acquired identity as a poet, while still making it clear that she also fancies him sexually as a bit of rough-and-ready. He is after all that walking contradiction, partly truth but mostly fiction, a peasant-poet. Looking back over his literary life from the asylum, Clare described it as being 'one chain of contradictions' (*LP*, 1, p. 45). The expectation that he would remain a peasant, while still being a poet, was the most important link in this particular chain.

The scene then shifts to the fields outside Holywell. The governess is lying in wait for the poet, lingering in his path, as he begins his walk back. She talks again about poetry and the need to start a correspondence. Clare is after all now a man of letters, of sorts. He apparently tries to get rid of her, but she is enjoying playing the part of patroness to a peasant-poet too much to halt her performance of it now. She may be a marginal figure herself at the big house, and yet now she can command the attention of somebody whose own awkwardness and marginality led him to mistake her for a real lady. It beats the governess trade. After they have walked and talked for a long time, they are apparently interrupted by the sudden, melodramatic entrance of a man on horseback. The governess dives for cover, mistaking this intruder for the General himself, the ultimate figure of authority. She carries on her conversation with Clare after this false alarm and it was only when 'it grew between the late and early' (*AW*, p. 126) that he manages to get away from her. He did not apparently want to get involved with her. He had been married for about a month. His wife, Patty, was heavily pregnant at this event and some of the evidence suggests a shotgun wedding to prevent patrons from associating him too closely with the perceived vices of the working classes. He eventually wrote the governess a cold letter that gave no room for a reply: 'there the matter or mystery ended for I never unriddeled its meanings tho it was one of the oddest adventures my poetical life met with' (*AW*, p. 126). He suspects that the governess had fallen in love with him. He identifies her as a poetry groupie, whereas she seems to see herself as a patroness as well. She is not named and the only further information about her identity that is supplied is that she comes from Birmingham (where the Reynardsons had property), a place that apparently did not promise much for Clare as it did not as well for Austen's Mrs Elton.

Clare's account of this drama at Holywell was probably loosely based on fact, even if the later parts of it appear to be laced with laddish fantasy. But the story as story, the play as play, does not have to be true, whatever that means, in order for it to capture in heightened form some of the central features of his literary life. Indeed, he seems to be using a few of the events of the day as starting points in an attempt to try to read, retrospectively, the riddles of this life as it confusingly began to unfold. As suggested, mistaken identities hold the key to some at least of the mysteries of Holywell Hall as well as to Clare's career more generally. To put it at its simplest, once he had been identified as a peasant-poet it proved impossible to shake off the label or brandname despite the quality and quantity of his work.

Clare almost wrote a poem about Holywell Hall. As it is 'Hollywell' describes his journey there rather than doing the sensible thing and praising his patron (*EP*, 2, pp. 42–6). It is all about travelling rather than arriving. 'Hollywell' celebrates the pleasures of strolling, or soodling, off the beaten track. The poet meanders idly through the landscape, stopping from time to time to lean over a post or loll against a tree. He leans and lolls, lounges and lingers, and then resumes his lolloping walk across the unenclosed heathland. He passes on slowly and almost furtively, as startled as some of the animals and birds that he himself surprises. As Ronald Blythe puts it, he is the 'master of the startled moment'.[6] The 'fluskering pheasant' and other birds can fly without restrictions here: no cages. Memories of childhood are touched and triggered by a sight here and a sound there. Despite being written in clip-clop couplets, the poem itself still soodles along, lazy and lingering, ambling and rambling. The point of the journey, the 'doubtful fancys' of patronage waiting at the end of it, can be all but forgotten. The poet saunters through the landscape, hanging and hovering there perhaps out of a reluctance to allow this personal and poetic secluded space to be encroached upon and then enclosed by patronage. First of all the General and then the governess threaten to invade this solitary space, to transform it and the secretive poet, peeping John, who celebrates it into a mere commodity. The poem resists their attempts by ignoring them. Yet one of the riddles that Clare will have to try to solve is that his own poetic celebrations of the soodling solitary, one of his favourite voices which he used as well in 'The Village Minstrel' and many other poems, also inevitably invade the very spaces that he seeks to protect from prying and patronising eyes. Perhaps particularly in his poems about birds and animals Clare celebrates the secret, solitary and secluded. He nestles down and hides in order to observe other fugitives from the cruel and predatory human world. And yet he himself is also, whether he likes it or not, still part of this world, as are his readers.

The rest of this chapter will be primarily concerned with establishing the identity, or part, that the General and his kind expected Clare, the peasant-poet, to play by considering the patronage of some other poets who were marketed and merchandised in broadly similar ways. They were expected to be ever so grateful to be able to flutter and warble away for a short time in the glass birdcages provided by their extremely generous patrons. As will be seen, this suited some who were content just to use poetry as a convenient means for material ends. Yet others found themselves painfully restricted by being expected to assume an identity or character that denied opportunities for development, difference and growth. It was like being placed in a straitjacket, or waistcoated, in a lunatic asylum, and the waistcoats there were very definitely not smart, 'dandyish', black ones. These other life stories are being told because they illuminate Clare's own one.

Mary Wollstonecraft uses the image of the gilded birdcage in *A Vindication of the Rights of Woman* (1792) to show the way in which marriage imprisons women. They might appear to be majestic as they stalk from perch to perch pluming themselves and building nests, but this majesty is mock and therefore mocking. Publication gave writers like Clare a voice, while at the same time trying as well to deny them one. This was the confusing mystery of Holywell Hall which Clare had to spend the rest of his literary life trying, with varying degrees of success, to unriddle.

As noted, *Poems Descriptive* was successful, transforming Clare virtually overnight into an object of curiosity and, according to his version of the Holywell drama, desire. The central features of his literary life, defined just for the moment in narrow terms in relation to publication in book form, was that he was unable to repeat this success. This was not in the script, no matter how hard he tried to take over the story and write his own play of his own life. His second volume, *The Village Minstrel*, which contains a more conventional celebration of Holywell Hall, was published in 1821 and attracted relatively little interest. Clare is once again described as a Northamptonshire Peasant on the title-page. After a very long and dispiriting delay a third volume, *The Shepherd's Calendar*, was eventually published in 1827. This did not sell at all well, even when Clare took the unusual step of hawking the unsold copies around his neighbourhood. He became a pedlar of his own poetry because the firm of Taylor and Hessey had already been disbanded on the grounds that poetry was no longer a marketable article. The bottom had dropped out of the market. Clare's last volume, *The Rural Muse*, dedicated to Earl Fitzwilliam, attracted some favourable reviews when it was published in 1835 but not enough to re-launch his career. This was the last-chance saloon. Taylor claimed that everybody thought that it contained the best material that he had written.[7] There is, however, no lottery more hazardous than literature, except perhaps prizefighting. Two years later Clare began the equivalent of a life sentence in lunatic asylums, dying in 1864. The glass birdcage of patronage that beckoned in 1820 was eventually replaced by another, but perhaps related, form of confinement.

Marketable articles

Robert Southey, the Poet Laureate since 1813, received a begging letter in 1827 from one John Jones, a rhyming butler straight out of a very bad comedy. Jones ever so humbly asked the Laureate for an informed opinion about some verses that he had penned in his limited spare time. Southey eventually decided to help him raise a little cash through publication to see him through the remains of his days. This was because he raised hopes about the existence of deferential members of the serving classes at a time when such reassurances were desperately needed: the First Reform Act was eventually passed in 1832 after a period of extra-parliamentary political agitation which often led to violence. An autobiographical letter, asked for to give Jones the opportunity to write his own reference (or 'character' as it was known as in this period), called Southey 'Sir' over thirty times. No one could possibly accuse him of not knowing his place. A place could therefore be found in 1831 for a slim volume, published by subscription by John Murray, still one of the leading publishing houses despite the break with Lord Byron, at a relatively expensive price. It was entitled *Attempts in Verse, by John Jones, an Old Servant; with Some Account of the Writer, Written by Himself: and an Introductory Essay on the Lives and Works of Our Uneducated Poets, by Robert Southey, Esq., Poet Laureate*. The method of publishing by subscription, common for uneducated writers, will be considered later in this chapter, even though Clare himself never quite had to resort to it.[8]

Jones was ever so humble, good Sir, about the merits of his writing, refusing to let it disrupt his domestic duties. This faithful old retainer often had to retain a poem in his head for several days on end because he did not have the time to write it down. He did, however, acquaint himself with Shakespeare's plays as he found an edition of them in the dining-room of one of his employers and set about reading them, but only after he had done his duty and set the table first. When he was not able to read Shakespeare upstairs, he dipped into the Bible downstairs.

Jones was published because he read great works, even if he was quite plainly unable to write them, and had the good sense to approach a very great man. The Laureate still felt it necessary to mediate his voice by placing it after a long introductory essay on the uneducated poets, in which it is claimed, maybe with a huge if suppressed sigh of relief, that he was probably the last poet in this tradition since universal education would inevitably destroy the conditions that had produced it. Southey indulges himself, and his readers, in antiquarian nostalgia. His mediating essay deals with six writers: John Taylor, Stephen Duck, James Woodhouse, John Bennet, Ann Yearsley and John Byrant. He devotes most space to the first one, Taylor, who wrote in the seventeenth century and indeed appears to lose interest in some of the later writers.

Southey's perspective is also influenced by cultural nationalism as he tries to establish a specifically English tradition of uneducated, or to use the term preferred by modern critics self-taught, writing. This means that he can conveniently ignore Robert Burns, James Hogg and other Scottish writers. He therefore preserves his condescending, dilettante stance by not having to deal with writers whose reputations might well threaten the security of his own precious, but also precarious, professional position. He also selects 'our' English tradition to protect his own power as patron. He refers towards the end of the essay to Robert Bloomfield, but postpones a full discussion of this literary life. Clare is very conspicuous by his absence. Southey's intention is to deal with poets who did not get anthologised, so the exclusion of Bloomfield and Clare can be taken as a compliment. Yet the aloofness of Southey's manner and his truly patronising tone were always in danger of turning it into an extremely backhanded one.

A detailed consideration of Bloomfield would have forced Southey, at the very least, to have recognised the fact that allegedly uneducated writers often outsold more established ones. *The Farmer's Boy* (1800) sold around 26,000 copies, going through seven editions in three years (as well as pirated ones in Ireland and elsewhere). It became the talk of the literary town, favourably reviewed by Southey himself and others. Bloomfield, an agricultural labourer who had migrated to London and worked there as a shoemaker for nearly twenty years, briefly became a literary curiosity because of what were seen to be discrepancies between his life and work. He composed the poem in his head in a noisy, overcrowded garret and yet, to the surprise and wonder of literary gentlemen, it still employed an individualistic, discriminating language. The content as well as the form of the poem was ultimately reassuring because it endorsed social discriminations. Its hero, Giles, is content to labour cheerfully on an estate governed by benevolent paternalism. It follows pastoral conventions, while still domesticating them, by reserving its criticism for an allegedly alien commercial economy that is seen as threatening to undermine the hierarchical harmony of the estate and, by extension, the state itself.

Bloomfield may have reproduced rather than challenged literary conventions, although an element of challenge was contained in the very acts of composition and publication. This was one of the reasons why Clare himself was such a devoted fan of Bloomfield's work. He planned to write a life of the author of *The Farmer's Boy* and increasingly came to identify with the way in which his writings, after their initial popularity, were largely neglected. He wrote three sonnets on Bloomfield and other poems often contain allusions to his writings. John Goodridge usefully draws attention to one of Clare's sketches of a tombstone bearing the names of Bloomfield, Keats and Thomas Chatterton.[9] Reflecting on the careers of other neglected writers was one way of understanding and coming to terms with the riddles of Holywell Hall. According to one biography, Clare had a picture of Keats on the wall at Helpston.[10] He represents himself as dead in 'The Fate of Genius' (*EP*, 2, pp. 666–70), allowing an old sexton who dug his early grave to tell his story. This sexton draws attention to the fact that the villagers thought that a peasant who wanted to be a poet could not be quite right in the head. The poem was probably written towards the end of 1821, when Clare's great literary expectations started to show some signs of being beyond his reach. He pictures himself as being pulled in different directions by the conflicting demands of his patrons. Looking at the life stories of other working-class writers is not a way of deflecting attention from Clare's own story, but rather of getting closer to it.

Clare ruined Southey's nostalgia by remaining alive, if only moderately well. He had been ill, off and on, throughout the 1820s: although not mad he was certainly melancholic in a much more general, everyday sense. He was trying to publish a fourth volume, provisionally entitled at this stage *The Midsummer Cushion*, at the same time as the deferential Jones was being ushered onto the literary stage as this very curious relic from a bygone age. He was angry a little later on with some journalists who 'force it down the throat of the world that I am asking charity when I am only seeking independance' (*LJC*, pp. 586–7). He was cross that a false impression had been created that his patrons were doing all in their power to help him, feathering a rent-free nest for him at Northborough, the village that he moved to in 1832. The smallholding there was owned by the Fitzwilliam family, but Clare paid rent for it. Jones was only too happy to accept charity, thank ye kindly kind Sir, and therefore allowed Southey, and his readers, to reinforce the security of their own positions. Clare's struggle for literary and social independence, to 'stand upon my own bottom as a poet without any apology as to want of education or any thing else' (*LJC*, p. 604), offered a direct challenge to a professional writer like Southey. It was therefore ignored. Clare is possibly dropping into the slang of the Fancy or prize-ring here: bottom was an all-embracing term for character, courage and pluck. If you had bottom, you had the right stuff. Alternatively, he may just be offering a shorthand version of the wise saw or proverb 'let every tub stand on its own bottom' (*LJC*, p. 589). He was not antagonistic towards Southey until the publication of Jones's poetry, beyond a bit of gentle joshing in the letters and prose writings. He draws attention to Southey's social pretensions in a knockabout poem called 'The Bards & Their Doxeys' (*MP*, 2, pp. 91–6), but then so did almost everybody else. It was a recognised literary sport. Clare had been impressed however by the Laureate's biography of Admiral Lord Nelson and Mark Storey finds echoes of one of Southey's Oriental tales in his poetry.[11] He responded, however, to Jones's volume (if it can be described as such) by noticing the contemptuous, 'sneering' (*LJC*, p. 538) manner in which Southey dealt with uneducated writers and the education question. The term uneducated writers oozes condescension. Clare also pointed out that, to add particular insult to general injury, Jones may have had the nerve to plagiarise one of his own poems (Bloomfield had also been ripped off much more systemically). To make matters even worse, the poem in question was about a bird. Clare is usually regarded as one of the best, if not the best, writers on birds.[12] Taylor diplomatically tried to look on the bright side, claiming that it was much better for Clare's reputation not to be included in Southey's 'dull Register'.[13] Charlotte Brontë was to receive a dusty answer from the Laureate in 1836 telling her that women had no place in the profession of literature. It was in Southey's interest to pick real losers like Jones rather than winners like Clare and Brontë.

Clare's more general criticisms of the volume were endorsed by some reviewers. The *Edinburgh Review* suggested in 1831 that Southey was primarily concerned to present writers who exhibited a 'reverence for antiquity, for social distinctions, and for the established order of things' (14, p. 76). The biographical sketches showed how these writers educated themselves, and were educated, into a deferential acceptance of dominant cultural assumptions. Ignorance of these was not considered to be a virtue. Primitivism and its potential for subversion held no attractions. Apparent exceptions were used to prove literary rules. The idea was to turn potential threats into pets.

Southey includes only one woman writer, Yearsley, in what still claims to be 'our' national tradition. Once again, he ignores the existence of writers (Mary Collier, Elizabeth Hands, Mary Leapor) who might have at least questioned his own credentials as a literary professional, although his claim to be primarily concerned with poets who were not anthologised is meant to provide some protection against such criticisms. He has enough trouble as it is incorporating Yearsley into his dilettante scheme of things. She had achieved popularity in 1785 with the publication by subscription of *Poems on Several Occasions by Ann Yearsley, A Milkwoman of Clifton*, which went through a number of editions. She had been discovered by Hannah More, known at this time as a poet and playwright rather than as the writer of counter-revolutionary tracts designed to suppress the alleged vices of the working classes. Although More's successful public relations offensive sometimes gestured towards forms of primitivism, she like Southey was mainly concerned to emphasise the way in which this particular uneducated poet had in fact educated herself into a justness and correctness of literary taste.

Yearsley, like Clare, did not want to be a one-hit wonder, or a one-trick pony. She had ambitions, later partially realised, to be an independent, professional writer working across a range of genres. Such dangerous desires could not be contained and confined within the glass birdcage of dilettante patronage. Yearsley and More engaged in a very public quarrel over access to the money that had been raised through publication. More believed that the working classes ought to be treated as children who would squander money in an improvident manner unless forcibly restrained from doing so by their betters. She felt that Yearsley was much too fond literally and more metaphorically of dressing up in showy clothes: becoming an upstart crow in borrowed plumage. She therefore set up a trust fund that was designed to benefit Yearsley's children at some unspecified date in the future. A number of Clare's letters in the late 1820s and earlier 1830s are devoted to trying to unriddle the rules governing his finances. He was also very fed up with the construction of an infantile, childlike identity for uneducated poets, implicit in the very term itself. Referring to his published books and the reviews of them, he asserted that 'if they cannot go without leading strings let them fall and be forgotten' (*AW*, p. 150). Leading strings, or what are called today reins, is a graphic way of describing the cultural mediation that was deemed to be necessary for poets who were seen as being beyond the literary pale, or off the beaten cultural track. Women writers often described husbands as attempting to keep their wives in leading strings: Lady Delacour in Maria Edgeworth's *Belinda* (1801) plunges herself into fashionable life as a way of resisting 'leading-strings'.[14] As to be expected, Southey comes down very heavily on More's side in his brief description of the quarrel. Her benevolent intentions, and by implication his own, should not have been so wilfully misunderstood.[15]

Southey, the professional man of letters, with justification prided himself on his understanding of the literary marketplace. His antiquarian tendencies did not prevent him from being very skilled indeed at public relations and marketing. He suggested that a self-taught writer called Henry Kirke White was able to achieve posthumous success because of the interest generated by his tragic life and death: 'For poetry is not a marketable article unless there be something strange or peculiar to give it a fashion; and in this case what money might possibly have been raised, would, in almost every instance, have been considered rather as given to the author than paid for his book'.[16] Kirke White was the son of a small tradesman from Nottingham. He began work at fourteen on a stocking-loom and yet succeeded in publishing a volume of poetry, dedicated to the Duchess of Devonshire, as well as in gaining a place at St John's College, Cambridge through a combination of self-help and patronage. He died in his college rooms in 1806 at the age of twenty-one. One of his contemporaries at the same college was a poor Irishman called Patrick Brontë. Next door at Trinity College there was a flashy young chap called Byron who was leading a very different lifestyle from these poor scholars: falling in love with a choirboy and apparently keeping a pet bear to annoy the fellows. He was also indulging his enthusiasm for pugilism and fencing. They were next door to each other, but also worlds apart. This also describes, as will be seen, Clare's relationship with Byron who nevertheless, to be fair, admired some of Kirke White's work when he found out about it.

Southey, the literary undertaker, decided that he could raise money for this particular dead poet's family through the publication of *Poetical Works and Remains of Henry Kirke White, with a Life by Robert Southey* (1807). He liked to work his own name into titles, as has already been seen with Jones's volume. Southey's commercial instincts were correct: the first edition sold out relatively quickly and had to be reprinted several times. The story of Kirke White's literary and scholarly aspirations appealed to gentry and middle-class readers. His remorseless and relentless pursuit of knowledge under difficulties also allowed him to become an important role-model for generations of working-class readers and writers, as evidenced in their autobiographical writings. His premature death added poignancy and therefore marketability to his work. It also just happened to mean that there was never any danger that he might upstage Southey as a writer.

Clare was given a copy of *Remains* in 1820, and was familiar with Kirke White's story before this. He describes the Reverend Isaiah Holland, a dissenting minister who was one of the first people to take his writing seriously, as being 'excessively fond of Kirk White' (*AW*, p. 45). An early sonnet contrasts his own isolation with the way in which Kirke White had been given a helping hand by the 'charitable' Southey (*EP*, 2, p. 382). Other writings from this time such as 'Solitude' (*EP*, 2, pp. 338–50) are influenced by Kirke White, as noticed by both Taylor and his flirtatious patroness, Eliza Emmerson, figures who will be discussed later.[17] Just as Clare himself came to interpret his own literary life through the experiences of writers from broadly similar backgrounds, so those who promoted him were also very conscious of some of the precedents and therefore identities that already existed. Drury's correspondence with Taylor, prior to the publication of *Poems Descriptive*, was concerned amongst other things to establish what lessons in marketing could be learnt from the careers of Burns, Bloomfield and Kirke White. While Drury's interest was mainly opportunistic, Clare's concern about and for these writers was much more passionate and personal. He identified with them. He was aware of Kirke White's story and imitated Burns's songs, as indeed he was to do later in the asylum. Their stories were, and are, his story.

Southey had already co-edited a volume of Chatterton's poetry in 1803 before he gave the reading public his account of Kirke White. This was an act of literary philanthropy to raise money for Chatterton's sister. Chatterton came from a poor background in Bristol and had died in Holborn, possibly by his own hand, in 1770 at the age of seventeen. According to the myth, his failure to find patronage killed him. Clare subscribes to this view (more modern accounts wonder whether Chatterton's attempts to cure himself of venereal disease might have been responsible for his death). Clare wrote an early poem on the death of Chatterton to some extent in the idiom of Chatterton (*EP*, 1, pp. 325–7), and continued to reflect upon a career that seemed to capture almost too perfectly and poignantly the riddles of literary reputation. Chatterton's name may have been well known amongst the people, but as a result of 'mellancholly memorys' (*AW*, p. 83) of his early death rather than because of a true appreciation of the quality of his work. Clare returns to this theme in his essay on popularity, which was published in *The European Magazine* in 1825, still trying to unriddle the mysteries of Holywell Hall. Almost all writers in this period saw possible reflections of themselves in Chatterton. Samuel Taylor Coleridge wrote a 'Monody on the Death of Chatterton', which Clare admired, and Keats dedicated 'Endymion' (1818) to the marvellous but tragic boy-poet. De Quincey dreamed about Chatterton's death. Clare was to copy Chatterton by attempting to palm off poems that he had written onto earlier authors: an act of literary insecurity as well of security.

Joseph Blacket's early death also helped to establish his marketability. He was a London-based shoemaker whose wife had died in 1807, leaving him to bring up a small daughter. The fact that he sought solace in writing poetry in the wake of this domestic tragedy meant that he could be presented as a deserving case for charity. His enthusiasm for established authors endeared him further to dilettante patrons. He died of consumption in 1809 and his *Remains* was published to raise money for his daughter.

Enter Lord Byron again, cynical as ever, to greet *Remains* with the mischievous thought that if 'Poor Joe' had in fact been published before he had died 'the wonder had been less, but the cruelty equal'.[18] This plays a playful variation on the themes of *English Bards and Scotch Reviewers* (1809), in which Byron, real scholar and gent, taunts patrons and the reading public more generally for allowing wonder, curiosity and gossip to become substitutes for literary merit. Clare was annoyed at his high-handed treatment of Bloomfield in this poem. Byron's position is as usual completely and utterly riddled with contradictions since his own gossipy style celebrates the very objects of his satire. He may have affected to be the scourge of marketable literary articles, yet this hardly prevented him from fashioning his own life and work into best-selling commodities. For those like Keats and Clare who struggled unsuccessfully to achieve literary independence, Byron's truly phenomenal success, internationally as well as nationally, became both inspiring and daunting. As will be seen, Clare started doing Byron impersonations as well as ones of Regency boxers during the asylum years. At one level, the neglected poet imprisoned in a Victorian institution assumes the identity of one of the most popular writers of the Regency period who courted success by seeming to shun it disdainfully. Here was another riddle. It was one that Clare had learnt to read. He described how an artist whom he knew 'affected to be little taen with worldly applause and was always fishing for it –' (*BH*, p. 138). This was Byron in very minor key. At another level, the rejected poet imprisoned for the rest of his natural life in institutions assumes the identity of a wandering cosmopolitan exile and outcast.

Clare happened to be in London in July 1824 (his third visit there) when Byron's funeral procession set off on its four-day journey to Nottinghamshire. Many of the carriages were empty: in death as in life there were those who did not want to be associated too closely with Byron and his scandalous reputation. Although Clare had read about the event in the newspapers, he was still surprised to see crowds of people gathering as he was soodling along Oxford Street to see one of his patrons. He joined them. It was only when 'a young girl that stood beside me gave a deep sigh and utterd poor Lord Byron' (*BH*, p. 157) that he realised what was happening. The scene he paints could have come from an Elizabethan theatre. Toffs look down from windows, seeing nothing but a spectacle that is being performed exclusively for their benefit. It is only the groundlings on the street who feel raw emotion as the procession bears the people's poet away. Clare's account and others indicate that Byron was one of the rock stars of his day. There was also a niche in this poetic hall of fame for members of the suicide society or crazy club like Chatterton, just as there is one today for the likes of Kurt Cobain.[19] Would Clare himself ever make it big time, or was he doomed just to attract the attention of literary folkies as a peasant-poet? Nobody in the crowd recognises him. He attends the event by accident. Perhaps this particular riddle in the fame game is that most stars are not really born until they die, by which time, of course, it is too late, at least for them.

Byron gleefully took every opportunity going, and some that were not, to sneer at the way in which Southey's early radicalism in the 1790s had been rapidly replaced by reverence for the established order of things. This was a familiar enough lad's game amongst writers such as Percy Shelley and Hazlitt, and radical publishers such as Richard Carlile. Byron's satires may, however, also have contained elements of self-satire. Both he and Southey were, unlike Clare, extremely skilled players of the literary market. The obsessive crusade and tirade against Southey may have been motivated by a more purely literary rivalry that recognised similarity as well as difference.

The reading public, unlike Byron, was prepared to be charitable towards literary curiosities like 'poor Joe' Blacket provided that certain rules were observed. Entitlement to charitable status usually had to be clearly announced in the title itself. As has already been seen, deserving cases were packaged up and labelled as such: 'A Northamptonshire Peasant', 'An Old Servant' and 'A Milkwoman of Clifton'. *Simple Poems on Simple Subjects, by Christian Milne, Wife of a Journeyman Ship-Carpenter in Footdee* was published by subscription in Aberdeen in 1805 and dedicated to the Duchess of Gordon. Before Milne married, she had been a domestic servant and had managed, like Jones, to acquire some knowledge of polite culture by reading books owned by her employers on the quiet. Secrecy, or inventing cover stories, characterised her whole educational history since her own family considered even basic reading and writing to be signs of idleness, signs no doubt of Satan. Clare was forced to invent less elaborate cover stories to prevent his parents from finding out that he was a writer. Milne's poetry nevertheless found its way into the hands of members of the local literary establishment, who encouraged her aspirations because they appeared to reinforce rather than undermine her sense of domestic virtues. She herself, rather than her writing, was the marketable article or product.

Readers are made acutely conscious of Milne's social status before a word of the poetry can be read, just as they were made aware of what Clare did for a living. The strong, double emphasis on simplicity in the title immediately allows a position of cultural superiority to be adopted. The foregrounding of her place of residence was intended to make sure in this particular case that local readers patronised a local writer. Directions are also being provided for literary tourists who wanted to visit her to check out her charitable status for themselves, as happened with her as it did with Clare. When volumes were published in London, however, as was the case with Clare's ones, the identification of locality can perhaps be seen as the way in which a metropolitan literary culture may define itself and its 'Other'. Having said this, it is still important to remember that Clare became a Cockney of sorts.

The patron's text

Writers who allowed themselves to be marketed by dilettante patrons and philanthropists were usually prevented from addressing their readers directly. Their work was carefully mediated and framed by introductions, prefaces and footnotes composed by their patrons. It was felt that they could not possibly even toddle without these 'leading strings'. As has been seen, titles, usually chosen by patrons, were texts in their own right. Taylor chose Clare's first three titles and also suggested ones for publications that did not materialise. Clare was pleased with the choice of *Visits of the Early Muses* for his '*old* Poems' (*LJC*, p. 383). Eliza Emmerson was responsible for the title for his fourth volume. An extreme example of this process of cultural mediation occurred in 1773 with the publication in London of *Poems on Various*

Subjects, Religious and Moral, by Phillis Wheatley, Negro Servant to Mr John Wheatley, of Boston, in New England. Great care was taken to establish the authenticity of this particular article since it was believed that the wide discrepancy between social position and cultural achievement might adversely effect its marketability. The reader is offered different kinds of documentary evidence before being allowed to read the poems themselves. A drawing of Wheatley in the act of composition is followed by a statement from her master which reassures readers that they are buying a genuine article. This is followed by a signed guarantee from eighteen eminent Bostonians that Wheatley is who she says that she is. Genuine was a term that was often included in the titles of works by uneducated, or self-taught, writers to reassure potential purchasers. It also crops up in similar publications by discharged and often wounded servicemen, those suffering from physical disabilities and many others who felt that they had a legitimate one-off claim to the benevolence of the reading public. Taylor's introduction to *Poems Descriptive* invited those with any doubts about the genuineness of this particular article to come and stare in wonder at the manuscript at his shop.

Framing and mediating devices were a common feature in religious conversion narratives in the Regency period, so it is not surprising to find them also being used extensively in what were essentially literary conversion narratives. The apparently chance discovery of approved literary works, so the story goes, leads Jones, Milne and many others towards the literary light of polite culture. Taylor made much ado of Clare's entry into polite culture through the purchase of James Thomson's *Seasons* (1726–30). Clare eventually bought this in Stamford and climbed into Burghley Park to read it on his way home. The peasant was on his way to becoming a poet.

Mary Saxby's *Memoirs of a Female Vagrant, Written by Herself,* published in Dunstable in 1806, was edited by Samuel Greatheed. He prefaces the *Memoirs* with a letter about his editorial policy to one of her patrons, in which he justifies the omission of material that is not strictly related to the theme of religious conversion. His prejudices against vagrants, apparent in the very choice of the term itself, are clearly visible throughout the letter. There is not the remotest glimmer of the fascination that Clare felt for gypsy life, lived as it was at the unenclosed edges and margins of society. Saxby is therefore allowed to speak only within the narrow confines established for her by her editor. Her narrative, when it is finally and grudgingly given permission to speak, is frequently peppered with editorial footnotes, which are designed to make sure that not even the very simplest soul misses the moral of the story. She is almost being strangled with 'leading strings'. She is, for good measure, denied the last word as well as the first: when the narrative breaks off, Greatheed closes the volume with his version of her story. She is allowed a voice only to be ultimately denied it. The editing here is particularly high-handed, but it was a style that was also adopted by many other dilettante and philanthropic patrons in literary conversion narratives. These other narratives help to explain the way in which Clare was constructed as a writer.[20]

Poetical Attempts, by Ann Candler, a Suffolk Cottager: with a Short Narrative of Her Life was published by subscription in Ipswich in 1803. The narrative of her life was clearly meant to establish her as a member of the deserving poor. She had spent over twenty years in a workhouse, after she had been deserted by her drunken husband, a character who would have been at home (or not) in Wollstonecraft's *Maria, or the Wrongs of Woman* (1798), resembling as he does the husband in the landlady's tale towards the end of the novel, after Maria, Jemima and the baby have escaped from the lunatic asylum. The fact that, at one point during their stormy relationship, she had walked out on him was a potentially uncomfortable one for her patrons. This is perhaps why she represents her time in the workhouse as her punishment. Confinement, often in prison, is a dominant theme in many conversion narratives. The editor of the volume, probably Elizabeth Cobbold, stresses the way in which Candler was strengthened by religion as well as by literature during her confinement. This is why it is deemed appropriate to raise money for her through subscription publication. As with Jones and Milne, it was her humility, or 'unobtrusive good qualities', that made her a marketable article.[21] This was primarily another exercise in literary philanthropy.

As will be seen, women such as Eliza Emmerson and Marianne Marsh took a particular interest in Clare's literary life, following in very general terms the example set by Frances Dunlop's patronage of Burns and the Duchess of Buccleuch's help for Hogg. As noticed, a flirtatious governess apparently tried to patronise Clare at Holywell Hall. Literary philanthropy, although not an activity confined exclusively to women, was nevertheless still one in which it was legitimate for them to demonstrate organisational skills as well as literary sensibilities.

As noted, uneducated writers were often published by subscription. This was a method which involved individuals undertaking to buy copies of a book before it appeared. Their names were then listed within the book itself, sometimes at the beginning, and thus competed for attention with the author's own name. A popular volume could have a very long list indeed. The one for the second, or Edinburgh, edition of Burns's *Poems Chiefly in the Scottish Dialect* (1787) ran to 37 pages, its length causing some last-minute production problems. The list for Hands's *The Death of Amnon* (1789) ran to 32 pages.

Before Clare attracted the attention of Drury and then Taylor, he had been negotiating with a local bookseller called Henson to bring out a volume by subscription. Those with money like Byron could pay local booksellers, in this case John Ridge of Newark, to publish their work privately but this was never an option for Clare. Henson's target was 100 subscribers, but the list does not seem to have even made double figures. The advertisement suggests a title along the lines of *Original Trifles, on Miscellaneous Subjects, Religious and Moral, in Verse, by John Clare, of Helpston*. Henson (a dissenter who appears to have got into trouble with his congregation later on) was hoping to sell Clare on the basis of his piety as well as on his interest to local readers. His occupation is not thought to be a specific selling point for this readership at least as far as the title was concerned, although he himself drew attention to his poverty in an Address to prospective readers. Given his mixture of shyness and arrogance, this was a particularly hard thing for him to write. He found the whole of this experience with Henson acutely embarrassing: 'I detested the thoughts of Subscription as being little better then begging money from people that knew nothing of their purchase' (*AW*, p. 17). Bloomfield's death in 1823 prompted him to make another attack on publication by subscription, contrasting the fate of a true genius with the attention paid to hacks and hackettes with subscription lists 'belarded as thickly with my Lord this & my Lady tother as if they were the choicest geniuses nature ever gave birth too' (*LJC*, p. 301). The humiliation of his association with Henson comes to the surface again in 1825 when he notes the existence of 'about nine neighbour Poets who have printed their trifles by subscription' (*LJC*, p. 334). There is also a poem poking fun at the local competition (*MP*, 2, pp. 3–5). He has not forgotten that he himself was originally going to be presented to the neighbourhood as a writer of mere trifles. As will be seen, one of his patrons did establish a fund by subscription for him. There were times when he referred to it contemptuously as a begging list. Above all, Clare wanted to be independent and taken very seriously as a writer. He did not want to be trifled with.

An experienced publisher, which Henson was probably not, would have made sure that readers would have known what they were getting by publishing in advance the names of the leading subscribers to guarantee that this was a genuine article. Henson could of course reply: first catch your gentleman. He was hoping that a 'Dedication to a *Gentleman* will certainly help the sale'.[22] Drury suggested to Taylor this kind of advanced notice for Clare's first volume, arguing that the names of some of Clare's aristocratic patrons would encourage the gentry to flock forward as subscribers (his target was 300). This was common practice. After Yearsley's break with More, there were announcements in the local press indicating that she could still command titled patronage. Drury, conscious of the tradition of writing and publishing into which he wanted to place Clare, whose writings he described as 'the trembling and diffident efforts of a second Burns or Bloomfield', was still thinking in terms of publication by subscription.[23] Taylor's commercial instincts nevertheless favoured publication at the publisher's risk (known in the trade as on speculation) which was the method eventually chosen. Clare approved of this (*LJC*, p. 48). There had been a plan to dedicate the volume to a local Whig grandee, Viscount Milton, but this was dropped just before publication perhaps because he did not respond to the request. Taylor nevertheless seems to have been against the idea (*LJC*, p. 25). He is acting as a commercial publisher in voicing his suspicions of subscription lists and dedications to great men. As will be seen, the commercial publisher who believed in the market and one of the aristocratic patrons, Lord Radstock, who believed in conspicuous philanthropy, did not see eye to eye. Clare thought that dedication hunting was worse than fox-hunting. He had to put his reservations about publication by subscription on hold later on in his career as this seemed, initially, to be the only way that he could get a fourth volume published. With help from friends, he was able to collect about 200 firm promises of purchase, but was in the event able to sell the copyright (for forty pounds) instead.

Charlotte Richardson was a domestic servant from York who had two volumes of poetry published by subscription: *Poems Written on Different Occasions* (1806) and *Poems Chiefly Composed During the Pressure of Severe Illness* (1809). The money that she made from the publication of the first volume allowed her, after initial difficulties, to establish herself as a schoolteacher. There was never any question, or danger, of her becoming a professional writer. This was not in the script. Her success was the direct result of the patronage of Catherine Cappe, the widow of a prominent Unitarian minister. Cappe was a remarkably energetic philanthropist, who was actively engaged in campaigns for lady visitors to superintend the female inmates of such institutions as charity schools, infirmaries, asylums, workhouses and prisons.

Richardson had attended a Sunday school where, according to Cappe, she gave early signs of her potential to become a good servant by exhibiting qualities of 'quickness' and 'docility'.[24] She was then sent to the Grey Coat School, a charitable foundation that educated female paupers and orphans into their eventual roles as humble domestic servants, seen but not often heard. Her first experiences in service were harsh but, on the strength of a 'character' or identity from Cappe, she was able to obtain a better position. Increased wages allowed her to buy some works of polite culture, and this is where the literary conversion narrative kicks in. Cappe nevertheless takes pains to stress that reading did not interfere with this maid's work. Like John Jones and Christian Milne, she knew her place.

Most servants lodged with their employers and were expected to leave when married. Richardson became ill again almost immediately after her marriage. She still had to look after her sick husband, who eventually died of consumption in 1804. It seemed as though her small son was in danger of going blind, so she tried to provide for both of them by starting a school. One of Cappe's philanthropic friends just happened to call on her shortly after the death of her husband and found her trying to express her grief through writing a poem. This was shown to Cappe who was immediately 'struck with the piety of the sentiments, affected by the pathos with which they are expressed, and utterly astonished at the neatness, not to say elegance of the composition'.[25]

Cappe had come to prominence as a philanthropist in the 1780s as a result of her successful campaign to reform the Grey Coat School. Although the sincerity of her concern for Richardson is not in question, her literary philanthropy clearly had its self-regarding aspects. She was after all promoting herself when she promoted the poetry of a former pupil of this school. Her name appears in the full titles of both of Richardson's volumes, and she claims the authority more generally to speak for the author in her two biographical introductions. Her own publications are advertised at the back of the first volume. Richardson, like other writers in this tradition, was in danger of being denied a voice at precisely the same time as she was being granted one. She too was almost being strangled with 'leading strings'.

Cappe selected the poetry itself and exercised considerable control as far as the second volume was concerned when, to be fair, Richardson may have been too ill to have had much involvement. The poet who is brought to the attention of charitable readers sings the praises of the professional and philanthropic members of York society and of the various institutions with which they were associated, including a lunatic asylum called the Retreat which will be visited in a later chapter. Although the patron's text is being defined here for convenience as that which was actually written by patrons themselves together with the subscription lists, this is clearly a narrow definition. It can be argued that these sort of songs of praise belong as much to the patron as to the poet. Indeed, publishing uneducated writers was a form of Regency vanity publishing as far as the patron was concerned. Cappe provides footnotes to many of the poems. These supply yet more biographical information, fill out and sometimes correct theological points and, more generally, underline the morals of the various stories. Poets and patrons often quarrelled over notes, as happened for instance with Bloomfield's *The Farmer's Boy*, but there is no evidence of any disagreement here. Although Cappe may not have paraded Richardson's ever so humble origins in the shortened titles of the volumes themselves, her editorial style was based on assumptions about her own superiority. She plays the mistress, kindly but somewhat severe, while the poet remains cast in the part of a humble servant, thank ye Ma'am.

The poems were published locally, yet Cappe's formidable organisational skills ensured that they also reached a wider audience. She wrote a long circular letter to influential national periodicals telling the story of her discovery of Richardson's poetry and announcing that a volume of it would be forthcoming. Henson was not in the same league as her, although Drury was approaching it. There were, originally, no plans to publish a second volume of Richardson's poetry, perhaps because to have done so might have been regarded as presumptuous. A short shelf-life was part of the script. Literary curios had a brief walk-on, walk-off part. It was a speaking part, although improvisation was ever so strictly forbidden. This was the part that Clare was expected to play and yet he refused to do so because he knew that he was a writer.

A few subscribers to the first volume agreed to pay much more than the asking price. The Duke of Grafton, one of Bloomfield's main patrons, put his name down for five guineas and was put on a separate, more exclusive subscribers' list. He believed in conspicuous philanthropy: patrons should be clearly visible on stage rather than tucked away more discretely in the wings. Regency society was obsessed by nuances of precedence, or what Austen sometimes referred to as consequence, making the subscription list a fascinating text in its own right. It was usually arranged alphabetically, although very occasionally it was ordered by rank. Alphabetical lists drew attention, however, to the rank and title of particular individuals as well as to the amount of money subscribed. Like the guest lists for exclusive parties that were published in the newspapers, they provided a strong sense of social standing, of who was really who in a particular locality or else within the wider literary community. Subscription lists figure prominently in a wide range of other publications. Lunatic asylums and other institutions dutifully listed their benefactors every year. General Birch Reynardson was on the list for the Lincoln Asylum.

Subscription lists played endless variations on the snobbish game that Southey played when introducing his faithful old retainer. He dwarfs plain John Jones not just by reminding everybody that he himself is Poet Laureate still, but also by insisting somewhat bogusly that he is also a gent by adding Esq. (or esquire) to his own name. It was not just lords and ladies, admirals and generals, bishops and clerical magistrates who paraded their titles for all to see. The monstrous regiment of real and wannabe gentlemen was also determined to get in on this particular act in the overall drama. Clare notes that many subscribers to worthy causes pay their guinea just so that they can be described as esquire in the newspapers.[26] He found himself on a subscription list by mistake in 1830 and quickly set the record straight (*LJC*, p. 503). A number of the villains in 'The Parish' proudly and pretentiously call themselves esquire: 'The meanest tradesman in his flash attire / Struts from behind his counter an Esqr' (*EP*, 2, p. 741). Being denoted as esquire signified coming of age as well as real or wannabe social status. Austen (whose name appears on the subscription list for Frances Burney's *Camilla* (1796) along with that of Maria Edgeworth) wrote to one of her nephews after his eighteenth birthday to say how delighted she was that she could now use this grown-up mode of address.

Cockneys and peasants

Keats was given a very brutal review in *Blackwood's Edinburgh Magazine* in August 1818 by John Gibson Lockhart, a Scotch reviewer who was Walter Scott's son-in-law. This was the fourth in a series of attacks on the Cockney School and was particularly vicious when it came to the politics of names and naming, or name-calling. It was a piece of bare-knuckle literary pugilism. Keats, a trained apothecary, is urged to use his own medical skills to cure himself of an infection, or addiction, for poetry and then return to his genuine social identity behind the shop counter: 'It is a better and a wiser thing to be a starved apothecary than a starved poet; so back to the shop Mr John, back to "plasters, pills, and ointment boxes" &c' (3, p. 524). Keats is being named as a mere tradesman might be: he may be mister, but he is still also a child who can be called just by his first name. He is still in leading strings. Earlier on, this review accuses him of 'insanity' and 'imperturbable drivelling idiocy' (p. 519).[27] It did not pull its punches.

Clare credited Keats with 'classical accomplishment' which, despite his overall admiration and identification, he felt could be too intrusive.[28] Keats in return admired Clare's work but, like others, felt that it could be too descriptive. Keats's enemies had a vested cultural interest in trying to deny that anybody from his background could possibly appreciate Classical literature. The Cockney School, which was taken to include Leigh Hunt (dubbed the King of the Cockneys by Lockhart) as well as Keats, were seen as vulgar upstarts and interlopers who did not know their place. Hazlitt, the great hater, was to join this hate-list. Lockhart describes Hunt as being a plebeian, and therefore by implication an uneducated writer, who minces about posing, preening and parading as a man of letters. The Cockneys were quite simply too cocky by half: arrogantly strutting and fretting their second-hand stuff. If they succeeded, then even governesses and peasants would be encouraged to publish, according to Lockhart. The line had to be held. Their subject matter, which in Hunt's case included incest, was seen as being well beyond the pale of polite society in its seamy and steamy sensuality.

The hostility towards the Cockneys was clearly not just a literary matter. *Blackwood's* was a patrician bastion of high Toryism. Keats's own radical political opinions, and those that could be imputed to him through his association with Hunt who had been jailed for lampooning the Prince Regent and continued to champion liberal causes in *The Examiner*, meant that he appeared to be doubly dangerous.[29] As will become clearer, Taylor has acquired a somewhat sinister reputation in Clare criticism for the way in which he edited the poetry. What therefore requires emphasis is that he took Cockneys and peasants seriously as writers when this was a bold and courageous thing to do. Publishing Keats was always bound to be a risky venture and therefore a daring one. Taylor nevertheless insisted that some of the steamier passages in 'Lamia' had to go. He prided himself on having resisted the temptation to publish Byron on moral grounds, although he would not have gone bankrupt in 1825 if he had done so. He encouraged controversial authors such De Quincey and Hazlitt, and yet always had a strong sense of where to draw his own line. The *London Magazine*, which he took over in 1821, refused Hazlitt's apology for Guy Fawkes on the grounds that it was not safe to publish it, presumably so soon after the

Cato Street Conspiracy of 1820 had apparently threatened the government. Publishing Clare was not so fraught with the risks involved in publishing Cockneys given the precedents (the other life stories), and therefore safety-nets, that already existed. Yet, as will be seen, poems by a Northamptonshire Peasant no matter how carefully labelled and packaged were still able to generate controversy, published as they were at a time of acute political and cultural tension when the suppression of working-class vice was considered to be a vital concern by the ruling classes.

Clare was not strictly speaking a peasant in 1820 as he did not own and work his own land, although it was always his dream to be able to do so. Before awaking and finding himself famous in 1820, he had had a wide variety of jobs from an early age: thresher, ploughman, gardener, nurseryman, agricultural labourer and lime-burner. Employment was mixed with spells of unemployment and underemployment, as was common in work governed by seasonal demands. Clare's poor health did not help matters. Just before he was theatrically discovered by Drury, it is possible that his parents were only one short step away from the workhouse. The family was badly in debt and it is unlikely that, alone and unaided, Clare could have rescued it. He had also served in the militia, and was a writer a long time before he was discovered to be one, perhaps starting seriously in about 1808.

The description of Clare as a peasant was not meant to be taken too literally since his publishers were using the term as a brandname. It evoked images of sturdiness and independence, but crucially within an overall acceptance of a deferential society. A peasant, the backbone of a legendary, mythological old country called England, could therefore be safely patronised. The term also implied a degree, but an acceptable degree, of naïveté. The poems were seen as being descriptive rather than philosophical. They were simple rather than learned (shades of Christian Milne). Clare was sold as a peasant, and yet Drury warned him not to make too much of this background as he might be 'accused of discontent, ambition and the Lord-knows-what'.[30] His first two volumes were nevertheless accused of just some of these things. It was a no-win situation.

The brandname of peasant also set up expectations that Clare was part of a tradition of writing that merited attention, as much for philanthropic as for literary reasons, as Taylor stressed in his introduction to *Poems Descriptive* even though he was suspicious of aristocratic forms of patronage. The apparent wonder of Clare's discovery could be contained within another narrative that emphasised continuities and precedents (Burns and Bloomfield). This is one of the reasons why some of these other stories have to be told here. Few peasant-poets actually fitted the bill according to strict, as opposed to more symbolic, definitions. Those connected with agriculture were usually labourers like Clare rather than smallholders. Perhaps it was only Burns, whose reputation, as will be seen, was always higher than Clare's, who came close to answering the job description. Yet peasant-poets could in fact be domestic servants, labourers and artisans, particularly if they wrote on rural themes. Their precise occupation was not as important as the more generalised set of qualities, social as well as literary, that they promised to deliver. The terms eventually become interchangeable: 'uneducated', 'unlettered', 'humble' writers in 'humble circumstances' are also by symbolic definition peasant-poets.

Many writers in this tradition appear to have got what they wanted out of patronage and publication. Poetry proved to be a nice little earner for Jones, Milne, Candler, Richardson and many others. Those who died young were not in a position to complain about the restrictions imposed by the glass birdcage of patronage, or indeed about Southey's activities as a literary undertaker. In terms of the sheer volume of this kind of writing which solicited philanthropic concern from its readers in the Regency period, which can only be hinted at here, it was in fact only a minority of writers who beat their wings against the cage after finding it difficult to build a comfortable little nest within it. Yet these are the cases that are best remembered since they concern writers who were good enough to want to make a living out of writing rather than being content just to parade their living, or occupation, to compensate for the supposed deficiencies of their trifling, simple works. The argument has been that it is still necessary to recover some sense of the success stories, in material terms, of literary philanthropy in order to understand the careers of those writers like Clare who reacted against it and the narrow identity that it imposed.

The mystery that Clare had to start unriddling at Holywell Hall and later on was that, despite confusing appearances to the contrary such as the actual publication and favourable reception of his first volume, the dramatic script was written, and being updated throughout his literary life with new but still familiar scenes, to prevent him from becoming a literary professional. This was a closely and jealously guarded class and gender privilege, by Southey and other influential figures. Clare might, if he had acted his part correctly, have been found a job in the gardens at Holywell Hall. This, or something like it, had to be the limit of his ambitions. He could not become a literary superstar like Byron, Southey and Walter Scott, who was knighted in 1820. The ceilings imposed by dilettante patronage were very low, even if the fact that they were made out of glass sometimes made this difficult to spot. This was another part of the riddle.

The clerical magistrate whom Clare was forced to ride over to visit in 1820 suspected all labourers of being no-good-boyos. A man overheard whistling while he worked was immediately branded as being in league with poachers, although he was in fact fencing and thus enclosing land. According to Clare, this magistrate 'mistrusted every stranger for thieves or vagabonds' (*AW*, p. 123). Clare was not a literary stranger in the sense that Burns, Bloomfield, Hogg and others had already been permitted to pass beyond the 'no trespassing' sign into the enclosure that was literature.[31] To use one of Clare's own images, writers such as Hogg and himself were like 'stray cattle' (*LJC*, p. 303) who had soodled into the field of literature. But nobody really knew just how far Clare could be trusted to be there. Was his identity that of a harmless enough peasant-poet who could be safely patronised until the next one inevitably wandered in with his or her trifles, or would he suddenly and dramatically reveal himself to be a poacher-poet who was going to steal the jealously guarded possessions of the literary professionals? Was he a thief and a vagabond? Hogg, known as the Etterick Shepherd, reacted to the perception that he might be 'an intruder in the walks of literature' by claiming that he was 'only a saunterer, and malign nobody who chooses to let me pass'.[32] This saunterer nevertheless just happened to produce *The Private Memoirs and Confessions of a Justified Sinner* (1824), which has rightly claimed much more attention than anything else written by the *Blackwood's* group. Until relatively recently some critics were still not prepared to accept that a mere Etterick Shepherd could have penned this haunting and perceptive account of the psychology of evil, and so attributed it, or at least parts of it, to Lockhart instead. A similar thing happened to Clare. After the publication of *Poems Descriptive*, a number of people in the locality claimed that he was just a front and that the volume must have been written by Drury or somebody else.

Clare was often caught, sometimes perhaps trapped, between different worlds. He spent some time in the upstairs world at Holywell Hall, before going to eat his meal in the downstairs one. He spied on a suspected poacher with the magistrate, before going back to Helpston to the company of poachers and gypsies. When travelling by coach to London for the first time in 1820, he was not sure whether he was actually meant to be on the coach, or labouring in the fields that it passed through: 'I coud almost fancy that my identity as well as my occupations had changed that I was not the same John Clare but some stranger soul had jumpd into my skin' (*BH*, p. 134). Such examples could be multiplied. There is also a sense in which Clare was caught between different literary worlds. One world, which has been examined here, was a place in which old-style dilettante and philanthropic patronage, together with subscription lists and other 'leading strings', still reigned supreme. Reports of the death of old-style patronage around the middle of the eighteenth century have been much exaggerated. It continued well into the Regency period and was deemed particularly appropriate for humble poets. Yet there was another emerging world in which commercial publishers like Taylor, readers and the market played more active parts. One way of reading Clare's literary life is to see both his life and works as becoming battlegrounds on which these different literary worlds either clashed, or else negotiated uneasy truces. This at least is a proposition that can be explored more fully in the next chapter. Taylor himself was also caught between these two worlds: he invited curious readers to come and stare in wonder at Clare's manuscript and yet he also treated him very, very seriously as an important writer with his own voice.

2
That Man I Would Have Him To Be: Public Relations and Peasant Poetry

Hot blood

It is roundabout nine in the evening on 16 February 1821. It had promised to be a bright, moonlit night but by now the fog is coming down and rolling around. Two men ride up to the Chalk Farm Tavern, out Hampstead way. They give their horses to the ostler and go inside. They are twitchy and do not stay long, saying that they will be back to finish their drinks in a while. The servants at the tavern know exactly what game is afoot since Chalk Farm is duelling country: the equivalent of the Bois de Boulogne in Paris where Mr Rochester, a Regency rake whose name also harks back to excesses of the Restoration period, fights a duel. It is only a matter of time before pistol shots are heard ringing out.

The ostler dashes in the direction from which the shots have come. A man rushes into the tavern, shouting out that a friend of his has met with an accident. He and some of the servants grab the window-shutter that was always kept handy to be used as a stretcher on such occasions and run to the scene of this accident. They find a man there, lying on his back covered with a coat and a military-style cloak. He is writhing around in agony, having been shot through the groin. Two men are huddled together in conversation some yards away.

The wounded man is brought back to the tavern with difficulty: the ostler grabs his shoulders and others hold his feet to prevent him from falling off the shutter. Somebody is sent to fetch his own medical man. There had been a surgeon and his apprentice present at the duel, palely loitering behind a hedge wondering if they were going to be needed. He has already given his opinion on the duelling ground that the wound is probably a mortal or fatal one. He is right, although the wounded man still takes ten days to die. He appears to recover when the bullet is removed, but then relapses. The inquest starts at the tavern on the evening of 1 March. A verdict of wilful murder is eventually returned against the other duellist and the two seconds who had been involved. A subscription fund is established for the dead man's family.[1]

Despite the unambiguous nature of this verdict, it is still not entirely clear what happened on that foggy night. It seems likely, however, that both duellists had deliberately fired either wide or high with their first shots (known in the jargon as deloping), even though this may not have been clear at the time. This was quite common, providing a cue for claims that honour had been satisfied to be proffered and accepted, followed by an adjournment to the tavern to seal the peace. There were some occasions when no shots at all were fired. This happened earlier at Chalk Farm when the poet and songwriter Tom Moore, a best-seller in the Regency period but not much read now, challenged a critic to a duel over a bad review. The seconds deliberately delayed the proceedings long enough for the forewarned Bow Street Runners to arrive in the proverbial nick of time. There was some doubt over whether the pistols ever got properly loaded, which allowed Byron who prided himself on being a good shot to make a rude joke about Moore's leadless pistols and lack of balls. Moore attempted to challenge Byron to a duel as a result of these remarks. One of the hinges around which Tom Stoppard's play *Arcadia* (1993) turns is whether or not Byron himself fought in a duel with a minor (fictional) poet. Clare may have been hoping to emulate Moore's success when he allowed, against the advice of his publishers, some of his poems to be set to music. Although duels could degenerate into farce as here, they were often deadly serious affairs. About seventy people were killed in duels during George III's reign (1760–1820) and it seems likely that there may have been some unrecorded deaths as well. Very senior politicians, far from seeking to discourage this practice, fought in affairs of honour (sometimes with each other) just like other members of the duelling classes.

Something seems to have gone wrong after the first shots had been fired at Chalk Farm. This may have been the result of poor visibility which prevented both sides from realising that this was meant to be a duel of theatrical gesture rather than one of murderous intent. This in turn was probably made worse by the inexperience of the participants. This may have been the first time that they had been called out. Whatever the reasons, it appears that the second of the man who was to receive the mortal wound urged him to fire his next shot for real. It was fatal advice. The other second also seems to have lost his cool.

If the duel not fought by Tom Moore was close to farce, this one with its swirling fog and men wrapped up in military cloaks was absolutely pure melodrama.

The trial was fixed to take place at the Old Bailey on Friday, 13 April, a date that did not augur well for the defendants. The court was packed two hours before proceedings were due to begin. The second who had given the fatal advice did not put in an appearance. He had been holed up in France, but was now under cover in London. He was tried later. The two other defendants, who had also been in hiding in France and then in London to avoid arrest, were dressed in mourning: a nice theatrical touch. That Regency rotter Sir Mulberry Hawk escapes to France after killing somebody in a duel in Dickens's *Nicholas Nickleby* (1838/9). A Bow Street Runner called Davis had in fact put in an appearance at the Chalk Farm Tavern shortly after the duel there but, with the kind of apparent incompetence that would have exasperated Dickens, had allowed the participants to disappear into the foggy night. Perhaps some money had changed hands.

The confusing events of that foggy February night were pieced together with help from the medical men, the ostler and the landlord of the Chalk Farm Tavern. The defendants, both of whom were lawyers, did not give evidence (probably for fear of incriminating themselves) but were allowed to call a large number of character witnesses. These included an MP, the master of an Oxford college and several lawyers. It was then time for the judge, who had sentenced the Cato Street Conspirators to death the previous year for High Treason, to direct the members of the jury. He reminded them that, if the event was premeditated, they ought to bring in a verdict of murder. At first sight there did not seem to be any doubt that this was indeed the case. The surgeon and his apprentice were not exactly there by accident. But the judge suggested that the fatal second shot may still have been fired in anger, in hot rather than 'cool blood' in legal-speak, after the etiquette of the duelling ground had been broken.[2] If so, then this meant a verdict of manslaughter. Before bringing this in, the jury needed to consider the excellent character statements that had been given by the great and the good, as well as the fact that the defendants would punish themselves for the rest of their lives over what had happened. Although it seems that the judge was steering the jury none too subtly towards a verdict of not guilty, this is not how it appeared to the duellist who was on trial. His letters both before and after the trial indicate that, at the very least, he feared the charge of manslaughter might stick. He must therefore have been mightily relieved when the jury came back after about half-an-hour and declared that the defendants were innocent. On the same day at the Old Bailey a petty burglar and an inept mugger were sentenced to death. The greatest crime against property was indeed to have none, and then to try to get your grubby hands on the possessions of others. As Byron put it during one of his speeches in the House of Lords, poverty was seen as a capital crime by those who made the law.

The man who eventually died as a result of this duel at Chalk Farm was John Scott, the first editor of the *London Magazine*. He was, somewhat ironically, in the middle of a series of articles on living authors at the time. He had just written one on Byron. The man who shot him, apparently in hot blood, was Jonathan (Henry) Christie who was associated with *Blackwood's Edinburgh Magazine*. The trashing of Keats by Lockhart in this journal provides some of the background to the events at Chalk Farm. Keats had died in Rome on 23 February, while Scott was still struggling for his own life. Yet Scott had also been annoyed at the way in which Lockhart and his cronies made very personal attacks on other English writers. Coleridge and Hazlitt were amongst those who were rubbished (despite the fact that Coleridge wrote for *Blackwood's*).

According to some accounts it was Hazlitt, who enjoyed a good fight and disliked most things Scottish, who pushed Scott towards the duel. Hazlitt, known to the *London Magazine* group as 'our Mr Drama' as a result of his theatre reviews, could certainly be a histrionic drama queen at times. Clare, who liked his critical writings but not some of his political rants, pictures him as severe, sneering and suspicious. He was particularly active immediately after Scott's death, filling up the magazine with his own articles as well as those that he had persuaded friends to write. Some thought that he would become the new editor but his contributions, which included 'Table Talk' as well as drama and art reviews, tailed off when Taylor took over during the course of the summer.

Reviews were usually anonymous in this period. Clare sounds off against 'the cold hearted butchers of annonymous Critics' (*LJC*, p. 188) when reflecting on Keats's death. It needs to be emphasised that he felt part of this metropolitan literary scene. Authorship was often, however, an open secret. Scott and Lockhart were trying to identify each other as the enemy by clearing away some of the fog that was floating over this particular literary duelling ground. Scott wanted to know the precise nature of Lockhart's association with *Blackwood's*: was he an editor or not? Lockhart, using Christie as a go-between towards the end of the quarrel, wanted Scott to apologise publicly for remarks which it seemed could be attributed to him. The *London Magazine* was often frothy and frivolous, camp and comic. The duel nevertheless provides a reminder of the dark side to literary politics.

London fields

The *London Magazine* entered the literary lists in 1820, defining itself to some extent in opposition to *Blackwood's,* which had been in the field since 1817. The Edinburgh publication had its resident peasant-poet in James Hogg. Although the dialogues called *Noctes Ambrosianae* in which he appeared in caricature form did not start until 1822 (allegedly based on convivial gatherings at the Ambrose Tavern), his associations with Lockhart and the other members of this Edinburgh school of night were well known before this. It may well be that the *London Magazine*'s enthusiastic adoption of Clare (and later of Allan Cunningham, who joined up in December 1820) needs to be seen as part of the rivalry between the two journals: anything Hogg can do, Clare and Cunningham (who had in fact been poached from *Blackwood's*) can do better. Perhaps, more generally, the acquisition of a peasant-poet meant that *Blackwood's* would find it harder to claim that the Londoners were essentially suburban in their sympathies. James Hessey had written to his partner Taylor back in 1818 to say that *Blackwood's* needed to be taught a lesson: 'It is really time these fellows were put down.'[3] The *London Magazine* tried to do just this.

There was a profile of Clare in the very first number, immediately prior to the publication of *Poems Descriptive*. It was done by Octavius Gilchrist, a writer from Stamford with a particular interest in Renaissance literature, and prominently placed as the second article. Gilchrist recounts his first meeting with Clare, before going on to describe the poet's pursuit of knowledge under extreme difficulties. He takes some care towards the end of the profile to distance the Northamptonshire Peasant from forms of religious dissent, underplaying the early patronage of the Reverend Holland and perhaps even of Henson. Clare is presented as a devout member of the state church whose 'modest demeanour and decent habits are every way creditable to the faith he has thus conscientiously adopted and adhered to' (*CH*, p. 41). Clare colludes in this cover-up. His 'Sketches in the Life of John Clare Written by Himself', written to supply his publishers with biographical details, contains a savage attack on religious dissent towards the end (*BH*, p. 30). Gilchrist's message was not the same one that Taylor had been picking up from Drury who was concerned that Clare, like Burns, was hitting the self-destruct button. This could be part of the part for male writers. The women ones, by contrast, were always expected to be docile and deferential, meek and mild. Clare was reported to have a fondness for women and drink, and an aversion to hard work. Drury claimed that he would be 'afflicted with insanity' if he continued to mix his addiction for poetry with his addiction to drink.[4] Gilchrist's profile, which bends or spins the evidence to make Clare more acceptable to readers, established a pattern that others were to follow.

Clare was very much part of the literary group that gathered around the *London Magazine*, even though he was geographically apart from it for much of the time. The point requires stressing, since some still want to see his literary life as being in some way unique, untouched by mainstream literary history. He was, however, packaged in the same way as other peasant-poets had been. He was associated with a particular publishing house and a literary magazine. He met most of the contributors and, as will be seen, wrote perceptive pen-portraits of them. His marriage was announced in the magazine (1, p. 482). *Poems Descriptive* was reviewed by Scott, who was impressed, as later critics have been, by the particular sense of place that was displayed (1, pp. 323–8). There was another profile of Clare in 1821, this time by Taylor, just before the publication of *The Village Minstrel* (4, pp. 540–8). Taylor defends Clare's use of provincial language. Clare contributed regularly to the magazine, when Taylor eventually took it over after Scott's death, under his own name and more occasionally under that of Percy Green. He wore a green coat during his visits to London. The character was a parody of a peasant-poet although, given the way in which such poets were constructed in the first place, it could be seen as a parody of a parody. He also parodied the parody with another character called Stephen Timms. Some of Clare's contributions to the magazine were unattributed, meaning that he was more of a player in this game than is sometimes recognised. As mentioned throughout, Clare was a deeply ambitious writer and the *London* appeared to offer a way of realising this.

Clare is one of the writers, Londoners as well as others, whom Keats's friend J. H. Reynolds hauls up before the literary police office at Bow Street in a comic piece in 1823. He is playfully accused of having seduced one of the muses. He pleads poverty but does not escape being fined: 'Clare is said to have a wife, and ten little children all under the age of four years which makes his case more reprehensible' (7, p. 158). This account of Clare as a Jack-the-lad figure is close to Drury's warnings.

The following year the magazine published a poem called 'The Idler's Epistle to John Clare' in which 'cockney Clare' is seen as very much part of the group (10, pp. 143–5). He is nevertheless strongly advised to go back to the country for the sake of his health. It is suggested that if he does not, then he may end up killing himself. This and the other warnings that he received about his self-destructive lifestyle suggest that not all the biographical evidence may be available. He cruised the bars, boxing venues such as the Fives Court and the Regency equivalent of strip joints known as French theatres. Perhaps the Londoners had other things in mind as well. He was familiar with Pierce Egan's best-selling *Life in London* (1820/1), sometimes known after its two main characters as 'Tom and Jerry', and may have used it as a guidebook to the underworld. It seems likely that there may have been some casual sexual encounters along the way.

Taylor and Hessey sent Clare copies of the magazine on a reasonably regular basis. He lent them out before getting them bound. His publishers also kept him in touch with news of the other contributors, even after they had severed their connection with the magazine. Hessey tells him about Hazlitt's final illness in 1830: 'his mind is quite as ill at ease as his body'.[5] Clare responded to this event by railing against the way in which true genius was always misunderstood. Taylor passed on the news about Lamb's death, to which Clare responded (*LJC*, p. 624). Clare's literary life has sometimes been seen as taking place in not so splendid isolation from mainstream cultural developments, and having more links with folk culture. This was not however the case, certainly between 1820 and 1825, when Taylor sold the magazine. Clare's connections with it can be seen not just through his own contributions and his contact with other contributors, but also through some of the reading that he was doing back in Helpston in the earlier 1820s. For example, the Londoners were fascinated by *Macbeth*. De Quincey's essay 'On the Knocking at the Gate in Macbeth' is just one of a number of studies of this play in the magazine. Clare shared this fascination and claims to have read the play twenty times. There were also a number of articles on Shakespeare's representations of madness. More generally, Clare was following one of the main agendas of the magazine in his commitment to reasserting the importance of earlier writers. The magazine was his university.

Scott was brought up in Aberdeen and worked as a clerk (like a number of the *Londoners*) before becoming a journalist. He edited *The Statesman* and then moved to *Drakard's Stamford News* in 1809. He went on to edit *Drakard's Paper* in 1813 (which was based in London) and *The Champion* in 1814 which published Hazlitt, Keats and Reynolds. It was here that Scott reviewed Austen's *Emma* (1815/16). It is likely that his connections with Stamford, where he had lived while editing the *News*, helped in his decision to promote Clare as the *London*'s very own peasant-poet. The papers that he had been associated with had a reputation for tackling controversial issues such as the moral character of the Prince Regent. The actual content of his editorials in his early days as a journalist was sometimes every bit as radical as those to be found in *The Examiner* and *The Political Register*, and yet stylistically he had a knack of making his views seem more moderate and moderated. He knew a bit about the law of libel. He appeared to be more concerned with attacking the Regent's advisers. The *News* had criticised the flogging of militiamen in August 1809 which landed John Drakard, as owner, in prison for eighteen months even though the article was written by Scott. William Cobbett had made a similar attack two months earlier with broadly similar results. *The Examiner* produced extracts from Scott's article, although the owners, Leigh and John Hunt, were acquitted by a London jury. The floggings were objected to on patriotic grounds.

Scott's patriotism and the sense of fair play that went with it allowed him to criticise radicals as well as the Tory government in the *London* for placing the country and its constitution in danger. It was sometimes a case of a plague upon both their houses, at other times a recognition that no party had a monopoly on the truth. This was a bold move to make at a time when most journals were in bed with a particular political party: the *Edinburgh Review* with the Whigs, the *Quarterly Review* with the Tories, and so on. The first number of the *London* carried a piece on 'Politics and Public Manners' which described the dismissal of one of Clare's patrons, Earl Fitzwilliam, as Lord Lieutenant of the West Riding of Yorkshire for criticisms of government policy after the Peterloo Massacre (1, pp. 99–106). Scott may have been suspicious of mass radicalism, particularly in its more advanced forms, but he took up Fitzwilliam's case in the interests of fair play.[6] Other issues that he brought to the attention of his readers included legal reform. He wanted to see a new code established in which relatively minor crimes against property (such as petty burgarly and mugging) no longer carried the death penalty. This had been one of his main platforms in *Drakard's Paper*, in which he carried on a running battle with the Lord Chief Justice. As editor of the *London*, he was also preaching some of the same patriotic messages as he had done at *The Champion*, in which he had claimed, on 10 March 1816, that Britain had 'unrivalled capital, unrivalled skill, unrivalled establishments, unrivalled facilities of communication and conveyance, unrivalled freedom and superior morals'. Throughout his journalism the French, either explicitly or implicitly, are always the enemy. Although he continued his criticisms of the Regent's/George IV's ministers, he was less of a political journalist at the *London* than he had been back on *Drakard's Paper*. He saw himself now mainly as a critic and a travel writer. He had developed into a good critic, capable of discerning new literary trends and with a knack of picking important new writers such as Clare.

Clare may not have known Scott personally, but he clearly respected his abilities as an editor, as others such as Byron did: 'I knew nothing more of the man then by his actions which tells me he had more honesty and honour then his enemey'. The enemy here is Lockhart (suggesting again that Clare felt part of these Regency literary squabbles) whom Clare denounces as a 'd----d knave & a coward & my insignificant self woud tell him so to his teeth' (*LJC*, p. 164). Lockhart is being threatened with a punch-up rather than with a duel.[7] Clare notices in 1824 that *Blackwood's* has been criticising Taylor (for allegedly writing a bad review of Sir Walter Scott) and comments: 'there is no more Editor Scotts at present to check them' (*BH*, p. 185). While Scott lay dying, Clare asked Taylor for the latest news before telling a story that proved once again that journalism could be a risky business in the Regency period. Drakard had been beaten about the head and shoulders with a strong stick by an angry aristocrat who seems to have objected to being accused of hoarding grain.[8] Clare knew Drakard, as a bookseller as well as a newspaper man, who used to let him have books and newspapers on tick. When Drakard asked him in 1829 to become more involved in local journalism, he replied that he was not in the same league as a journalist as John Scott and Cobbett (*LJC*, p. 490). He appears to have been paid for his occasional contributions to the local press by being sent free copies of the papers concerned. Drakard wrote to him in 1831 begging him not to lend papers to the whole village as this meant that nobody there needed to buy them.[9] Drakard stopped sending papers a few months later.

Clare's own politics have often puzzled critics, particularly those who want him to be more consistently radical than he was. His views, as articulated in a series of manuscript notes and elsewhere, are often remarkably similar to those advanced by Scott. He too prided himself on being able to have friends on both sides of a question, and often asserted the virtues of common sense, fair play and honest practice.[10] He attacked the self-interest and pomposity of all political parties.

These views were in place before he joined the *London Magazine*, but perhaps as a result of reading the Stamford press. Scott is a missing link in much Clare criticism.[11] There are a number of patriotic earlier poems which, although they do not disguise the facts of the Revolutionary and Napoleonic wars such as disability and discharge, leave no doubt about whose side Clare supported. Although there were breaks in the fighting, war dominated Clare's society from his birth until he was over twenty. He was, as mentioned, a militiaman and may have come close to joining up on a more permanent basis. The defacing of the landscape which, as will be seen, becomes one of his major themes was being driven by the pressures of a wartime economy: enclosure was just one part of this process. Just as it is important not to fall for myths that Austen does not represent the Revolutionary and Napoleonic wars, so it is also necessary to insist that Clare was not detached from such major national and international events in some timeless, rural backwater. There was no such place.

Periodical journalism was usually a boys' own game in the Regency period and the *London* was no exception to this general rule. Clare referred to the contributors as 'lads of rare promise' (*LJC*, p. 203) and 'the merriest set of fellows I ever met with' (*LJC*, p. 243). Mary Shelley had two articles published in 1824, although the memoir of Byron that she submitted in the same year was turned down as at least one had already been commissioned. She does not appear to have been a guest at the monthly dinner parties for contributors instituted by Taylor. Mary Russell Mitford, who later wrote quite perceptively about Clare, was also an occasional contributor.[12] De Quincey published a provocative piece in 1824 in which he asserted that women did not have the same powers of imagination as men. He asks why there was no Mrs. Shakespeare, not aware that the answer lies in the very way in which the question itself is framed (Virginia Woolf was of course to suggest later what might have happened to Shakespeare's sister). The existence of female genius was then debated in a couple of responses to it, but the issue did not catch light, perhaps because most contributors and readers agreed with De Quincey. Clare certainly did: 'Dequincey had a paper on "false distinctions" which contended quite right enough that women had an inferior genius to men' (*BH*, p. 182). As will be seen, this kind of misogyny becomes even more rampant at times in the asylums.

The atmosphere was masculine although, more specifically, the *London* provided a stage on which different masculine identities could be performed. Thomas Griffiths Wainewright (otherwise known as Janus Weathercock, Egomet Bonmot and Cornelius Van Vinkbooms) played, and indeed overplayed, the part of a very camp Regency dandy complete with pale yellow gloves and a blue coat.[13] He had failed as an army officer and was struggling as a painter, and had probably had some sort of breakdown just before he joined the *London*. He concentrated on theatre and art criticism. He was himself a theatrical work of art, eccentrically dressed with stage props which included a horse called Contributor and a Newfoundland dog named Neptune. He was by all accounts a generous host, cracking many a bottle along with many a joke. He invited Clare to dinner towards the end of May in 1822. Clare took a day or two to recover.[14] He describes Wainewright as a 'facetious good hearted fellow' (*LJC*, p. 494) and a 'very comical sort of chap' (*BH*, p. 146). The evidence suggests that this camp creation and the peasant-poet had a genuine liking for each other. They were both, in their different ways, conscious of playing a part. Their masks – Janus Weathercock and Percy Green – may have been disguises but they were also, as Oscar Wilde suggests in his essay on Wainewright, exaggerations or intensifications of their personalities.[15] They had interests in common. Wainewright championed Elizabethan writers like Christopher Marlowe and shared Clare's admiration for Isaac Walton. His criticism could be much ado about nothing: he had nothing much to say, but often said it entertainingly through a series of digressions and dialogues with other contributors, or imaginary readers. Funny things tended to happen to him on the way to exhibitions, or just when settling down to write articles. He was clearly influenced by Laurence Sterne. More or less everything was in quotation marks including the quotation marks themselves. Yet at other times Wainewright was ahead of the pack, for instance in his recognition of William Blake. Clare follows him: 'Blake was brave by instinct & honest by choice.'[16]

Wainewright joined the chorus of those warning Clare about his ruinous lifestyle when he visited London, even though he may have helped to lead the poet astray: not a particularly difficult thing to do. Clare's letters contain few jokes, obsessed as he was with his great literary expectations and his health. He nevertheless suggests to Hessey, tongue firmly in cheek, that they should ask Wainewright to 'create us one of his long legd beauties' (*LJC*, p. 283) as a frontispiece for *The Shepherd's Calendar*. Wainewright painted and collected naughty pictures. Not all the contributors were quite so amused by Wainewright's posing as a gentleman of letters. Hazlitt's essay on 'Vulgarity and Affectation' takes him to task, none too playfully, for his mannered, aloof and disdainful attitude towards popular culture, particularly popular theatre. He is described as a coxcomb.

Many of the Londoners aspired, like Clare, to be taken seriously as professional writers but very few of them were able to achieve this dream. The deck was stacked against Cockneys. It is possible that Wainewright, anxious to persuade everybody that he was a real gent, was not paid for some of his articles. The precedent here was Byron, another keeper of Newfoundland dogs, who loftily refused payment for his earlier commercial publications. Wainewright painted at least one portrait of Byron. There was family money, but Wainewright had difficulty getting his paws on it. This is why he began yet more careers, first as a forger and then as a poisoner. He, like the duellists and broken dandies such as Beau Brummell and Scrope Davies who had become busted flushes, spent time in France.[17] Discarded mistresses such as Mary Anne Clark, Dorothy Jordan and Emma, Lady Hamilton also fled to France, as did those such as Byron's daughter Medora Leigh who wanted to keep her pregnancy a secret. It was when Wainewright made the mistake of slipping back to England from France that he had his collar felt by a Bow Street Runner. He was eventually tried (for forgery rather than for murder) and transported in 1837 to Tasmania, which was known then as Van Diemen's Land, for the rest of his natural life. 1837, the date of Queen Victoria's accession to the throne, was a very bad year indeed for Regency relics. Clare began his life sentence in asylums then: both he and Wainewright had to survive hell on earth. Wainewright died ten years later, apparently hooked on opium, some of which he may have nicked from the convict hospital where he worked. Some dark demons lurked beneath the flippant, camp surfaces that he displayed in the magazine. Narcissism may however connect his apparently different selves. He was a Regency version of Dorian Gray, which helps to explain Wilde's interest in him: a connoisseur of evil as well as of beauty, or somebody who came to appreciate the beauty of evil.[18]

Reynolds was another contributor who was never able to establish himself as a professional writer, despite early promise. He continued to practise the law. Another articled clerk, William Harrison Ainsworth, was an occasional contributor. Barry Cornwall, who made more sustained contributions including ones on boxing, was also a lawyer. Later on he became a lunacy commissioner. Like Wainewright and Clare, Reynolds also found himself washed up in the early Victorian period, being described just before his death in the 1840s as 'discontented, broken down and habitually drunk'.[19] He cultivated the robust, rugged masculinity of the Corinthian man about town. In addition to theatre reviews, he wrote widely on boxing, wrestling and other sporting matters. He visited the Cockpit Royal for the magazine, which made even him a bit squeamish. Pierce Egan's young bucks also take in this sight.[20] Reynolds, like Hazlitt and others, connected the *London* to the worlds of bucks and bruisers, the Fives Court and the Fancy, turf and tavern. He had published a collection of poems in 1820 called *The Fancy* which purported to be the work of Peter Corcoran, a law student whose love of boxing proves to be his downfall. Corcoran was the name of a real boxer from the past. Reynolds was not the only wag who made connections between the poetic fancy and the pugilistic one. Clare and others were quick to spot Reynolds behind this particular mask (Taylor had sent him a copy of the book, parts of which he felt were nearly as good as Byron).

Reynolds was a big fan of a boxer called Jack Randall who was also, as will be seen later, one of Clare's heroes. In 1824 Reynolds did a long article under his usual pen-name of Edward Herbert on a notorious murder trial, the Thurtell case, which exposed the seamier side of the sporting world (9, pp. 165–85). Thurtell was a boxing enthusiast who had acted as second for one of Randall's opponents in 1821. He murdered a card-sharp and low-life hustler called William Weare who plied his trade at gaming hells and racetracks. Clare refers in passing to the trial in one of his letters, claiming that it had been eclipsed by the trial of the notorious Edinburgh body-snatchers Burke and Hare (*LJC*, p. 452). Some resurrection men had, incidentally, paid Helpston churchyard a visit earlier on. Reynolds's article about Thurtell is as much about himself and his journey to Hertford to watch the trial and his own reactions to it, as it is about the case itself. He was probably responsible earlier on for the promotion of Egan, the leading authority on boxing as well as on London low-life who had also covered the Thurtell trial. Reynolds claimed that Egan had actually helped Thurtell to prepare his defence. As *Blackwood's* had taken a shine to Egan, perhaps the *London Magazine* felt it needed to stake out its own claims to his writings. Egan's *Sporting Anecdotes* was favourably reviewed, probably by Reynolds. When Taylor took over after the death of Scott, he entrusted some of the editorial work to Reynolds.

The *London* had a medley of different contributors with their own agendas: the patriotic Scott hated Napoleon whereas Hazlitt worshipped him. Yet one of the things that united many of them (including Wainewright who enjoyed watching boxing, or rather watching himself watching boxing) was a desire to move effortlessly and knowledgeably between high-life and low-life, the overworld and the underworld. Crime and criminality fascinated the Londoners.[21] Clare was infected by these desires, although this is not always recognised by those who want to confine him to the folk tradition. He toyed with the idea of writing a 'low life' (*LJC*, p. 179) novel, perhaps encouraged by Egan's success. Taylor was supportive, despite the fact that he was not particularly interested in fiction. Clare describes Reynolds, with his hearty laugh and punning humour, as being the life and soul of the monthly dinner parties. He liked most of Reynolds's poetry although detected in it 'a good share of affectation and somthing near akin to bombast' (*BH*, p. 141). It is a perceptive description that could also be applied to some of the other Londoners, and indeed was by *Blackwood's*.

Lamb's Elia essays, which began in August 1820, were generally regarded as the magazine's star-turn. He was certainly usually paid more than the other contributors: twenty guineas per piece as opposed to the standard rate of ten. Like Reynolds, he remained in his day job, as a clerk in the East India Company, rather than risking the uncertainties of a career as a professional writer. Clare was by no means unique in having to combine writing with other forms of work. Real and adopted Cockneys were expected to know their place. Although Lamb had been mistaken for a Jacobin during the hysteria of the 1790s his stance, particularly as it developed, took the form of a much more generalised anti-authoritarianism mixed with a nostalgia which was quaint but also challenging. He and Clare may have differed over the nature of pastoral poetry itself, and yet they both offered celebrations of the customary calendar in particular and old customs more generally. Lamb's calendar was metropolitan, whereas Clare's was rural. Lamb was hurt by Southey's insinuations that his religious views were suspect and the title of his response, 'Letter of Elia to Robert Southey, Esquire', draws attention to the Laureate's social pretensions. Yet, although Lamb scores this and other points, his critique is mild in comparison with the full frontal attacks launched by second-generation Romantic poets like Byron and others. Like the other Londoners, Lamb attempted to embrace all aspects of metropolitan life. He suggests in 'A Complaint of the Decay of Beggars in the Metropolis', which Clare thought one of his best pieces, that fraudulent beggars should not be moved on by evangelical do-gooders but rather appreciated and supported as a form of cheap street theatre. Clare himself found it difficult to resist beggars so that, after giving them money, he 'was often as bad off as those I relieved' (*BH*, p. 149).[22]

Lamb's version of masculinity was often a remarkably feminised one. Wearing the mask of Elia, he represents himself as a mildly eccentric and idiosyncratic bachelor who needs his domestic creature comforts. He explains in 'Imperfect Sympathies' why he could never become a Quaker: 'I must have books, pictures, theatres, chit-chat, scandal, jokes, ambiguities, and a thousand whim-whams'.[23] Chit-chat, or gossip, is often the subject as well as the form of his essays. This whimsicality may well have been at odds with a domestic reality that was dominated by his sister Mary's intermittent madness (which will be discussed later). Like Wainewright, Reynolds and others, Lamb relished puns and other forms of wordplay. He declares in 'Witches and Other Night-fears' that, unlike Coleridge and, it might be added, De Quincey, he does not have a whole stud of nightmares. The mask may once again hide some of his own fears. The *London* reprinted in August 1822 an earlier piece, 'Confessions of a Drunkard', in which he addresses readers more directly. He describes how heavy drinking binges bring him to a precipice above the abyss of alcoholism: 'to mortgage miserable morrows for nights of madness'.[24] He was still taking out this almost daily mortgage when he met Clare. The poet describes how after an evening attacking the wine, Lamb, whose one concession to sobriety was to dress soberly enough in black, 'leans off' (*BH*, p. 142) into the night, always at risk of falling into the river on his winding way back home. At times Lamb may have been a cosy old thing, but at other times his lifestyle and attitudes flouted bourgeois respectability. His sister Mary highlighted the exploitation of needlewomen.[25]

Lamb's 'Confessions' may have been reprinted as a result of the popularity of De Quincey's *Confessions of an English Opium-eater*. The first part appeared in the issue for September 1821, which also contained a poem by Clare as well as Taylor's profile of him. The second part was published in October, with the book coming out the following year.[26] Clare asked his publishers to send him a copy of it as De Quincey was 'a great favourite of mine' (*LJC*, p. 269). He wrote two poems, 'Superstitions Dream' and 'The Night Mare', heavily under the influence of De Quincey, if not noticeably of opium. He thought at the time that the former was the best thing that he had written. Eliza Emmerson agreed with him.[27] As so often in his literary life, Byron is to be found lurking around in this case as another influence besides that of De Quincey. 'Superstitions Dream', which was published in the *London Magazine* (5, pp. 163–5), is about the Last Judgement and is full of yawning graves, crashing thunder and lightening, and the smell of sulphur as the devils come to claim their own. It is a powerful piece of writing which for modern readers has images that can be associated with nuclear Armageddon. Nature is wiped out and people are running around pointlessly in every direction. Then the sun just drops out of the sky:

> & oer the east a fearful light begun
> To show the sun rise not the morning sun
> But one in wild confusion doomd to rise
> & drop agen in horror from the skyes
> To heavens mid way it reeld & changd to blood
> Then dropt in darkness like a rushing flood
> (*MP*, 1, 329)

'The Night Mare' is about what appears to be a visit to heaven and Clare like De Quincey in his dreamscapes conveys an impression of almost endless space. It turns out however to be hell, complete with a 'foul fiend' with a 'horrid laugh' (*MP*, 1, p. 337). Clare is not a Romantic writer, yet he does have more things in common with some of the Romantics than is often recognised. Trances, reveries and dreams, whether induced by opium, drink or not, were regarded as heightened states of consciousness. The Book of Revelation was of course a major source for Blake and others. Clare may not have produced a stud of nightmare poems, yet at the start of his literary life as a published author he is, prompted particularly by De Quincey, clearly experimenting with some Romantic themes. As a prose writer, he was at this time also preoccupied with the story of his own life. The *London Magazine* helped to provide his agenda.[28]

Clare was realistic enough to recognise that the quality of the magazine was variable under Taylor's editorship, but felt that De Quincey and Lamb often held it together. Taylor and Hessey regarded the acquisition of De Quincey as a big coup since he was supposed to have become one of *Blackwood's* hired literary guns, but had created some bad feeling by not meeting his deadlines. Taylor lent him money so that he could complete *Confessions* and eventually paid him forty pounds for it. Whenever money changed hands, Taylor assumed that he had purchased the copyright although this was not always clear to some of his authors, including Clare. De Quincey received a very handsome advance for a project that was to come after *Confessions* which does not seem to have materialised. He nevertheless contributed to the magazine on a very regular basis. Like most druggies, his favourite subject was himself. He also contributed translations as well as essays on history, political economy and German writings. Scott had been keen that the magazine should deal with European as well as with British literature.

Clare describes De Quincey, despite his reputation as an opium-eater and formidable philosopher, as being remarkably childlike: 'A little artless simple seeming body somthing of a child over grown' (*BH*, p. 144). *Confessions* combines high learning with low-life in ways that fitted in with what has been identified as one of dominant themes of the *London*. Although De Quincey creates the impression that he is an alienated, wandering outcast who walks on the wild side of life and literary life, he had in fact the kind of financial safety-nets that were denied to Clare. His family paid something towards the tour of Wales that he undertook after doing a runner from school. He may have mingled with prostitutes like Ann(e) and slept rough when he first went to London, but he was not a complete down-and-out. He was there to try to borrow money from loan-sharks against his eventual inheritance. When he walks the city streets, he is usually very conscious indeed of his social as well as intellectual superiority. He came into money and went to university at Oxford for five years, amassing a large library. He rode the mail-coaches up to London in search of pleasure. Leaving university without a degree, he was able to live off his capital for a number of years. He established himself in the Lake District to be near his heroes, Wordsworth and Coleridge. He had money to lend (to Coleridge of all people!) as well as to spend on books, drugs and other creature comforts. It was only when his family money began to run dry that he was forced to try to earn a living by his pen, first as a newspaper editor and then as a writer. He was thirty-six when *Confessions* made his name if not his fortune. Cockneys came in different shapes and sizes. Although there are some general similarities between Clare's literary life and the careers of some of the other Londoners, there are also at times some significant differences.[29]

As a general rule, prose writers had a better chance than poets of surviving in the literary jungle. De Quincey eventually moved back to Edinburgh so that he could stay in close touch with *Blackwood's* and some of the other journals based there. Although prolific if still somewhat erratic over deadlines, he continued to lead a hand-to-mouth existence at least until his final years. Yet he was a full-time writer, unlike Clare who went back to working as a labourer at various points during the 1820s. Prose writers were more likely to get commissioned than poets, who were expected by many journals to send their work in on spec. It was possible for Regency poets to survive, even when the bottom appeared to drop out of the market towards the end of the 1820s, but this was easier to do if they had a number of strings to their bow. Letitia Landon, known as L.E.L., was a poet whom Clare generally admired. She was able to combine producing poetry with reviewing and editing, as well as with writing prose fiction. Clare's schemes for writing novels on such Regency themes as 'low life' and mail coaches did not get very far. A play in the idiom of Marlowe, one of Wainewright's heroes, did not suit him and was abandoned. There are, however, distinct echoes of Marlowe in later poems such as 'An Invite to Eternity'. Landon was able to base herself in London and thus maintain close and profitable links with journals such as *The Literary Gazette*.[30] This was not an option for Clare. He sent material to the annuals and almanacs that were becoming increasingly popular, but had no guarantees either that it would be accepted or paid for if it were. He complained to one editor that he had not been paid 'a farthing' (*LJC*, p. 458) for some of his contributions. He claimed to be owed six guineas. As Eliza Emmerson put it, these publications had 'a ready hand to *receive*, but not so to return that which is due'.[31] Clare got cross when he felt his work had been 'mutilated' (*LJC*, p. 350) by insensitive editors. He also contributed to local newspapers and, in keeping with his claim to have friends on both sides of a question, wrote for conservative as well as radical local publications. Yet there was not a living to be made out of such occasional forms of publication. As seen, payment may have just taken the form of copies of such publications.

Clare confessed that he was weary of writing for the *London* when Taylor decided to sell it off in 1825, although he was still disappointed by the way in which it had not lived up to its early promise. Lamb and other contributors also had mixed feelings about abandoning the sinking ship (or perhaps it was abandoning them). Clare once referred to the other contributors as 'the family' (*LJC*, p. 253) and later letters show him as being often desperate for any news and gossip about them. He made 'anxious enquiries' to one of the other Londoners in 1830 and got some news back about Lamb and Wainewright.[32] He tried to get Lamb's address from Hessey (*LJC*, p. 517). Allan Cunningham was the only one of the old gang who tried to stay in touch on something like a regular basis. The *London* did not, and could not, offer solutions to many of the riddles of his literary life and its chain of contradictions. If, however, it had continued for longer under either Scott or Taylor then it could be argued that he would have felt less isolated as a writer. Much has been written in Clare criticism about his 'sense of place' following John Barrell's work (and indeed that of John Scott).[33] This is an important theme, and yet it is just as necessary to insist that with the *London* group he found another kind of place which was just as crucial to his development as a writer. He does not deny this, even if some of those who claim to be supporting his work seem to do so.

The magazine has been described as 'one of the greatest literary periodicals that England has produced'.[34] Even though it included, as has been seen, some star-turns, this seems to be overstating the case. It also encourages comparisons with other historical periods, whereas the important thing about the *London* is that it was a quintessentially Regency production. Its heyday was during Scott's editorship with the quality becoming more variable under Taylor. The circulation was relatively small, around 1,600. To put this in some sort of perspective, the *Edinburgh Review*, which provided a platform for the wit of Sidney Smith, had a print-run of 13,000 in 1814. *Blackwood's* had a habit of exaggerating its circulation, but it certainly competed with the *Edinburgh*. A cyncial interpretation might suggest that Scott's attacks on Lockhart were part of a circulation war. Perhaps the lowish circulation of the *London* was caused by all the in-jokes and knowing comments about the real identities of the writers partially masked by their pen-names. Readers were of course given the opportunity to join this club or coterie, although at times the mannered, self-conscious nature of the writing seems to be erecting too many barriers. As Clare notes, there was a good deal of affectation and bombast. The Brontë children devoured *Blackwood's* and wanted to write for it. The *London Magazine* does not appear to have inspired this sort of passion, even though the later issues contained a witty piece at the front ('The Lion's Head') explaining why certain contributions had been turned down.

The medley of contributors means that it is easier to identify a general tone rather than specific agendas that can be attributed to the magazine. It had a raffish and at times louche air, particularly in some of Reynolds's contributions and in the attention given to Egan. It had one gloriously and obviously camp contributor in Wainewright and yet perhaps this was the tone of the magazine more generally (even though Scott himself disliked most forms of affectation). It was not just De Quincey who wrote obsessively about himself. Reynolds, Lamb and the others made their reactions more important than the issues and events that they were describing. The contributors appeared to be endlessly fascinated by themselves and their riddling, punning wit. They turned out in force for the monthly dinners to admire themselves and, if necessary, to laugh long and loud at their own jokes and the spontaneous puns that had nevertheless been so well-rehearsed beforehand in front of the mirror. Seemingly trivial everyday events and lives were treated seriously as well as mock-seriously. Narcissism, or enjoying watching yourself self-consciously performing an overstated part, ran rampant. The dandy (Wainewright), the underworld connoisseur (Reynolds), the political fighter (Hazlitt), the whimsical bachelor (Lamb) and the scholar (De Quincey) were all jostling each other for theatrical space. And then of course there was another camp, kitschy creation known as a peasant-poet, who wore a green coat together with a yellow waistcoat and silk cravat, and lived up to the image by drinking too much too often. Clare's literary life was intimately bound up with the *London Magazine*.

The squawk of flattery

Gilchrist's associations with Drakard, and thus with the radical end of Stamford culture, meant that there were risks attached to allowing him to introduce Clare to the literary world. He was considered by some to be a dangerous man.[35] Clare appears to have been somewhat in awe of him, usually addressing him as 'Sir' at the beginning of letters, whereas he adopts more familiar modes of address in his correspondence. Yet, as seen, his version of Clare in the event contained very little that could ruffle the feathers of members of the establishment. Some of the reviews of *Poems Descriptive* picked up where he had left off. There were local profiles, for instance in the *Northampton Mercury* on 29 January. That old warhorse *The Anti-Jacobin Review*, which knew a thing or two about sniffing out radicalism, declared itself satisfied that there was 'no envious spirit, no carping discontent' (*CH*, p. 105) in the poems. Not all the reviewers were quite so impressed. Lockhart (nicknamed Lackheart by Gilchrist) never knowingly passed up an opportunity to take a cheap shot at the *London*. He pronounced in *Blackwood's* that the volume (which he had not even bothered to read) had been puffed up out of all proportion to its merits and sternly warned Clare's patrons to make sure that he did not get ideas above his station. There was not much danger of that. One of Clare's patrons had written to Sir Walter Scott to try to secure a more sympathetic review in *Blackwood's*.

At this point Drury was probably still the person who knew Clare best of all and he, as has been seen, was acutely aware of some of the skeletons that were rattling around in the cottage cupboard. This is why the plans to train Clare as either a schoolteacher or a clergyman never got anywhere. Taylor emphasised to him that the 'strictest moral conduct' would be absolutely essential if he was serious about becoming a teacher.[36] Drury advised the poet to stick firmly to his resolution of avoiding 'swig', or drink.[37] Drury was a wheeler and a dealer who wanted to use Clare to hustle a bit of fame and fortune for himself: 'a trafficing hugster after self interest' according to Clare (*LJC*, p. 502). He described Clare as a goose that was capable, with careful handling, of laying golden eggs.[38] Yet his promotion of the peasant-poet may also have been motivated by a desire to challenge educational and other monopolies. He established himself as a campaigning journalist and a thorn in the flesh of the ruling oligarchy after he returned to Lincoln in 1822. Clare was promoted by people like Gilchrist, Drury and Scott who, although they distanced themselves from mass radicalism, were nevertheless involved in forms of civic reform. Their agendas, like that of the *London* itself, were liberal, reformist and patriotic. Taylor can be added to this list since, although he had been working in London for a number of years, still kept in very close touch with his provincial, market-town roots.

Drury knew that Clare was not a simple soul who was completely and utterly devoted to the state church. He tells Taylor that the Methodists were annoyed when Clare left them.[39] The poet had experimented with forms of religious dissent before his discovery and was to do so again in 1824. His heavy drinking was always going to be a time-bomb waiting to explode in the faces of patrons who wanted him to be both devout and deferential. He advanced the modest proposal at one of the convivial *London Magazine* dinners in 1822 that all the churches should be burnt to the ground and the parsons forced to beg for food.[40] Despite gallant attempts by others at damage-limitation, some of his patrons got wind of this envious, discontented and drunken outburst. They began to wonder if his religious views were quite as safe and sound as Gilchrist had suggested. Perhaps he was a dangerous and dastardly poacher-poet after all.

Taylor presented Clare as a deserving case for literary philanthropy in the Introductions to both *Poems Descriptive* and *The Village Minstrel*. He may not have had too much choice about this since the conventions of the conversion, discovery narrative were, as has been seen, already well established with readers. When Clare was finally given a chance to introduce his own work in the Preface to *The Shepherd's Calendar* he tried to distance himself from Taylor's literary philanthropy: 'I hope that my station in life will not be set off as a foil against my verses.'[41] Given the skeletons in the cupboard, Taylor was always going to be in danger of giving hostages to fortune when he insisted that Clare deserved philanthropic as well as literary attention. The poet's credentials were bound to be scrutinised very thoroughly indeed in 1820. Forms of surveillance were the order of the day. This was a time of particularly acute social tension, every bit as hysterical as the 1790s. The Peterloo Massacre was followed by the Six Acts, which attempted to close down radicalism as a popular mass movement by restricting the politics of petition, press and platform. The Cato Street Conspiracy was allegedly discovered soon after Clare's poems had been published (it had in fact been largely orchestrated by the government as a way of demonising radicalism) and the trial of Queen Caroline later on in the same year represented a very serious constitutional crisis which was exploited by radicals and others. There was not a British revolution, but there were few at the time who could be absolutely certain that this was not lurking just around the corner.[42] Clare appeared on the literary stage at precisely the same time as church and state seemed to be under considerable threat. His identity as a deserving case for charity, and more generally as a reassuring and comforting symbol amidst a sea of troubles, had to be carefully and thoroughly vetted. His credentials were probably scutinised more closely than those of other male peasant-poets. Admiral Lord Radstock, a vice-president of the Society for the Suppression of Vice (SSV), felt that he was uniquely qualified for this crucially important national task. He took on the case, with a vengeance.

SSV had been founded back in 1802. Although it is sometimes claimed that it grew out of the Proclamation Society which had come into being in 1787 with the intention of crusading for a reformation in manners and morals, this is not quite right. The two societies existed separately for a time with different, although occasionally overlapping, memberships. One difference was that SSV had a much higher number of women members. It is likely that Radstock was one of the people who brought the two societies closer together. He was also president of the Naval Charitable Society, as well as being actively involved in a range of other good works including being vice-president of an asylum. He was an aristocrat by birth being the younger son of an earl, which allowed him to try to pull rank on a mere tradesman like Taylor. His retirement if it can be described as such, which began in 1802, was spent fighting the good fight, through counter-revolutionary pamphlets such as *The Cottager's Friend* as well as through committee work against vice and immorality. He belonged to the Evangelical wing of the state church and had a powerful network of cronies in high places. He was Clare's best friend, and worst enemy.

Radstock had been Governor of Newfoundland from 1797 to 1800. As was customary, he spent only the summer months there. For those interested in prize-money like Austen's Captain Wentworth, this would have been a disastrous posting. The French did put in an appearance in 1796, but were then not seen again for a long time. The Governor was responsible for maintaining law and order, as well as for organising convoys to and from Britain. The main industry was fishing. Radstock had his work cut out dealing, if not with French themselves, then with some of those who supported their radical ideas.

The *Latona* had been involved in the full-scale naval mutiny at Spithead in 1797. It then sailed round to the Nore, apparently without a captain, to give support to the floating republicans there. Later in the same year it was in Newfoundland, perhaps as a punishment. As mutinies go, the one that apparently took place on the *Latona* on Thursday, 3 August was pretty tame and may not even have been recognised as such by veterans in these matters such as Captain William Bligh who lost control of other ships besides the *Bounty*. Some sailors refused to climb up the rigging and then turned a bit nasty when one of them was given a flogging. Radstock was determined, however, not to let things get out of hand. He had a division of the ship's company lined up on Sunday morning before the church service. He was taking no chances and so had the sailors surrounded by soldiers and marines. He did not mince his words. He began by announcing that the leader of the Nore mutiny back in England had been hung from the yardarm. The ringleaders on the *Latona* were then described as 'villains' and those that followed them as 'cowards'. They were all 'traitors' and could therefore expect no mercy. If there was the merest hint of any more insubordination and insolence in the ranks, Radstock's officers had orders to shoot first and ask questions later. They would be taking no prisoners. The gun battery in the harbour had been told to burn the ship with 'red-hot shot' at the very first sign of any further trouble. This meant more than just a whiff of grapeshot. Radstock's bullying tactics did the trick, which was just as well for him as the course of action that he was proposing was illegal on several counts.[43]

This crushing of the mutiny that never quite was did not put a stop to Radstock's troubles with radicalism. He noticed that Tom Paine was being widely read and so shipped in counter-revolutionary literature to be distributed to stem the tide of infidelity. As dangerous ideas were often fermented in pubs or over drink more generally, he proposed to his masters in London a tax on rum to raise money to pay for some of the costs of British rule. He had fought in the American War of Independence, but does not appear to have learnt any lessons from it. Others had, so his proposal was not approved. He also wrote to London with dire warnings that the local defence force, the Newfoundland Regiment, could not be trusted to be absolutely loyal to king and country because it contained too many Irishmen. His fears were justified as in the spring of 1800 a number of the Irish soldiers swore their allegiance to the United Irishmen, an underground radical movement. Five were promptly executed on a specially built gallows and others were shipped off to Halifax, Nova Scotia to await punishment. Radstock may not have been present when these sentences were passed, yet his actions as Governor suggest that he would have approved of them.

Radstock combined his obsessive crusade against radicalism with philanthropic concern for the poor of Newfoundland. He established a subscription fund for the relief of the destitute. He also raised a reasonably large sum of money for the repair of the local Anglican church. Age did not mellow him and, if anything, the reverse seems to have been the case. Clare was to see both sides of his character in action: an absolutely pathological hatred of radicalism, coupled with a quite genuine concern for those members of the deserving poor who did not have any ideas above their lowly station.

SSV had periods of inertia but was particularly active in the years 1819 and 1820, bringing a large number of successful prosecutions. Richard Carlile and his associates were targeted for publishing what were seen as being blasphemous libels including works by Paine, which had also been successfully prosecuted by the Proclamation Society back in the 1790s. Publishers became cautious. The first two cantos of Byron's *Don Juan* were published in July 1819, but anonymously, without the rude Dedication to Southey and with some misgivings by Byron's friends such as John Cam Hobhouse who were worried that the bawdy and blasphemy might offend. Hobhouse's caution may have had something to do with the fact that his own political opinions were to land him for a time in Newgate.[44] Predictably enough *Blackwood's* entered the fray and was offended, declaring that Byron was a foul fiend rather than a human being. John Murray eventually washed his hands of the project and the later cantos, from six onwards, were published by Leigh Hunt's brother, John. Byron, although no lover of Keats, found that the Cockneys were the only ones prepared to risk publishing him in unedited form. These sort of historical details, together with the fact that Byron's 'Memoirs' was burnt by his friends in 1824, are sometimes conspicuous by their absence in accounts of Taylor's cautious attitudes towards some of Clare's poetry.[45] Byron the aristocrat could and often did pull rank on the reviewers. Clare and his publishers were in a much more vulnerable position, not least because they were in England rather than out of reach in exile in Italy.

SSV was concerned with three main issues: keeping the Sabbath day holy by clamping down on trading and other activities; stopping the distribution of allegedly blasphemous and indecent literature and prints; and closing down what were known as riotous and disorderly houses. Although these were its main concerns, it also sometimes dabbled in cases that dealt with things like illegal lotteries, nude bathing and cruelty to animals. As the Society developed, it became more and more preoccupied with indecency. Like the government itself, it was dependent on tip-offs from busybodies and informants who had their personal motives and agendas, although this was of course often denied. Members of SSV, in common with other moral crusaders and vigilantes, often took an indecent interest in indecency. They were gratified at finding the vices they were supposed to be suppressing, as Sidney Smith noticed. Some of them became obsessed by the devious ways in which lewd books and prints were apparently smuggled into girls' boarding schools. Both Keats and Clare expressed macho irritation when Taylor tried to make sure that their writings did not offend 'boarding school Misses' (*LJC*, p. 112). Byron, although conscious that women readers had made his reputation (shining in boudoirs), declared defiantly when trying to get an uncensored version of the first two cantos of *Don Juan* published that he was not in the business anymore of making 'Ladies books'.[46] There was a swipe at the beginning of Clare's 'The Parish' at farmers' daughters who think that their education gives them a right to dictate poetic taste. Perhaps the poets may have been a bit out of touch about what these misses were reading. SSV helped to get the Vagrancy Law changed in 1824 to make it harder for hawkers of indecent literature to avoid detection. Although SSV claimed to be waging war against all forms of vice, Sidney Smith was right to notice in an article that named Radstock as a prime mover that its efforts were concentrated on low-income, low-rent vices that took place in public. Upper-class vice, particularly if carried on behind closed doors, continued largely unchecked. Prize-fighting which, although illegal, enjoyed aristocratic and gentry support was not targeted in a big way. SSV was deeply unpopular with radicals and many civic reformers, largely because of the way in which it operated so blatantly such double standards. Clare published a poem in 1821 in *Drakard's Stamford News*, which drew attention to the double standards involved in the policy of keeping the Sabbath day holy (*EP*, 2, pp. 518–19).[47] Radstock would not have been amused. When an Irish bishop was caught in a very compromising position with a strapping guardsman in the backroom of a London pub in 1822, radicals immediately branded him as yet another hypocritical member of the Vice Society, even though there was little evidence that he was one. It was, however, a good as well as a potentially damaging story.

Radstock was certainly a great commercial asset to Clare: his best friend. *Poems Descriptive* would probably not have quickly gone into four editions and sold nearly 4,000 copies without his networking. After checking out Clare's credentials or 'character' with the Vicar of Helpston and others, he launched his public relations offensive. He secured reviews in some of the leading journals by persecuting editors (according to Gilchrist), introduced the poems to his influential circle, started a subscription fund for the poet's benefit and gave him publicity in *The Morning Post*. Whenever Radstock visited a place, he made sure that the local library stocked copies of Clare's poetry. He knew a bit about the oxygen of publicity. A serious fall down some stone steps in April 1820 did not prevent him from promoting and publicising the Northamptonshire Peasant from his command headquarters in Portland Place in London. He tried to make sure that the grandees in Clare's neighbourhood did the decent thing. He was worried that the money (seventeen pounds) generously lavished, as he saw it, on the poet by the Fitzwilliam family at the end of a visit might be corrupting and so wrote to them to see whether they might be prepared to stump up a rent-free cottage. He wondered in another letter if they would like to employ Clare as a gardener, fixing his hours so that he would be left with some time to write. He wrote again on the same subject. It appears that the Marquis of Exeter's annuity for Clare was the direct result of an intervention by Radstock. Despite having virtually illegible handwriting, Radstock fired off letters to all and sundry who could help to promote his product. He also showered Clare himself with newspapers (sometimes five or six a week), counter-revolutionary literature, a dictionary and advice about subject matter. He did not know how to do things by halves. He campaigned for Clare in the same way that he had once maintained law and order in Newfoundland.

Clare, who prided himself on being (in the tradition of John Scott) a plain speaker and dealer, initially liked Radstock because, despite the huge gulf in social position, he exhibited the same direct, straightforward qualities. Clare was full of praise for his patron when he was writing his autobiography which he was hoping to be able to publish: 'there is a good deal of the bluntness and openheartedness about him and there is nothing of pride or fashion' (*BH*, p. 54). He goes on to contrast the virtues of real aristocrats with the vices of those who merely ape them, which plays a variation on the themes of his satire

'The Parish' which opposes newfangled vices with old-fashioned virtues. He ends his account of the Admiral, however, by noticing a certain naïveté and unworldliness about him. He was to claim later that he liked 'John Bull sort of fellows' (*LJC*, p. 429) because they did not need to be flattered. Radstock was most definitely an exception to this rule. He was not just a bluff naval cove like Austen's Admiral Croft. He was also a bully and an interfering busybody. There was a time when patron and poet were barely speaking to each other. It was almost like a lovers' tiff. Radstock demanded the return of his almost unreadable letters, just possibly out of a concern that Clare and his Stamford friends might publish them and embarrass him. They were apparently written, he tells Clare just before his death, in 'the most unbounded confidence'.[48] Clare found the frequent requests dating back to the beginning of 1821 for the return of the letters troublesome because, so he claims, he is unable to put his hand on them. Radstock was cross about this, as well as at the way in which Clare often took a long time to reply to his letters. (Clare was working again as a labourer, but this seems to have been forgotten.) Towards the end of 1821 Radstock was muttering darkly about Clare's 'unbecoming conduct' and 'chilling silence'.[49] The relationship had begun well, but had then quickly run into difficulties. At some point Radstock probably destroyed Clare's letters to him. Johanne Clare emphasises the need to understand the 'real and oppressive power' which Radstock expected to be able to wield over Clare as a matter of course at this particular historical moment: he had after all wielded the same power over the alleged mutineers in Newfoundland earlier on.[50] John Clare's 'Journal' indicates that at some point an uneasy peace must have broken out. When Radstock died in 1825 Clare described him as the 'best friend I have met with' (*BH*, p. 241).

The skeletons in the cupboard made a quarrel between patron and poet almost inevitable. It was, in summary, triggered by two things. First of all, some of the poems that appeared in the first edition were bound to offend Evangelical sensibilities at this time of acute social tension because of the earthiness of either their form or content. 'Dollys Mistake or Ways of the Wake' (*EP*, 1, pp. 532–5) tells the story of a girl who allows herself to be seduced after a day at the fair. 'The Country Girl' (*EP*, 1, pp. 115–16) is the story of a farm servant who falls for a young farmer who promises to help her escape to the town. 'My Mary' (*EP*, 1, pp. 78–82) is a jokey counter-pastoral (influenced by William Cowper) which emphasises the dirt and other unattractive features of rural life. By the time that the third edition was published, they had all been removed. They were no great loss, although Clare was particularly annoyed about the removal of 'Dollys Mistake', but then he was not always the best judge of his own work. He tells Hessey, for whom he seems to reserve his rare jokes, 'I think to please all & offend all we shoud put out 215 pages of blank leaves & call it 'Clare in fashion' (*LJC*, p. 84). Radstock objected to some of these poems, although his views were shared by Taylor and others. Drury reports Clare's initial reaction as being 'sturdily resolved to have no alterations'.[51] Here and later, however, he was not, as a Northamptonshire Peasant, in a position to argue the toss with aristocratic patrons.

Second and more importantly, Radstock had smelt out unacceptable radical views in 'Dawning of Genius' (*EP*, 1, pp. 451–2) as well as in a poem called 'Helpstone', modelled to some extent on Oliver Goldsmith, which was the first one in the volume. Clare follows a description of the cutting down of some trees with a very generalised critique of 'Accursed wealth'. Although it is seen as producing poverty and starvation, Clare's main concern is the way in which its scars and defaces the landscape itself: 'Thou art the cause that levels every tree/ & woods bow down to clear a way for thee' (*EP*, 1, p. 161). Earlier on he writes about trees being beheaded. This provides an example of the ecological awareness that has impressed a number of recent Clare critics.[52] Trees, ponds, wells and other features of the landscape are given histories, personalities and sometimes voices in Clare's poetry. The land, like the labourers employed to work it, is starving, exhausted and overworked. Its bones are being picked over. The land is like the labourers in some respects, but also detached from them in others. It is dying, being killed off by things such as enclosure which are represented as being crude and clumsy as well as cruel. In 'The Mores' (*MP*, 2, pp. 347–50) the plough is described as 'blundering' and the landscape after enclosure as being 'mangled'. In 'The Lament of Swordy Well' the plough is 'hasty'.[53]

Radstock demanded the removal of the offending passages and eventually got his way. Taylor, despite claiming that he was not as fastidious as the Admiral about smuttiness, colluded with some of the attempts to suppress vice in the poems, but was less happy (so he said) about this more overtly political form of censorship. Although he eventually caved in, he gave Clare some moral support: 'I like your independence, Clare, and am sorry that any persons should be so ill judging to screw you up to the squeak of flattery.'[54] Taylor is badly understating the case here: Radstock wanted to hear the squawk of flattery, very loud and extremely clear. As Taylor was aware, patrons had their own selfish agendas.[55] Publisher and poet could not afford, however, to make an enemy of a powerful figure like Radstock. As Clare put it, he had to knock under for his own advantage. Working at flattery appeared to be easier for him than having to go back to manual labour. Taylor mentioned diplomatically that the offending lines could always be restored when the storm had blown over.

It is surprising that Clare's self-appointed patrons did not demand the removal of a poem called 'Crazy Nell', which Clare thought at the time and for some time afterwards 'one of the best I had written' (*AW*, p. 103). This time he could have been right. It seems that Taylor may have been initially reluctant to publish it and had to be persuaded to do so by Drury. This may have been because it did not fit neatly into the image of the pastoral peasant-poet that was being constructed. Indeed, the reverse is the case since it casts Gothic shadows over rural society. Clare claims that it was based on newspaper story, although this has not come to light. He did take ideas from such sources, although here as on many other occasions his inspiration may also have been more purely literary. The crazy woman appears frequently in Romantic and other writings of the period, for instance in Wordsworth's 'The Female Vagrant'. There are also a number of visual representations such as Johann Füssli's 'Mad Kate' (1806/7). Perhaps there are also echoes in the title of Clare's poem of Cowper's crazy Kate, a character in Book One of *The Task* (1785), even though she is driven mad when her lover is killed at sea rather than after an attempted murder.[56]

At first sight it seems that the poem is going to be another of Clare's rather conventional narratives of sexual betrayal. It then turns into something much more disturbing. Nell slips away from home secretly one night to wait in the forest for Ben, who has promised to marry her perhaps in exchange for having sex with her. She is left there alone for hours. When Ben eventually turns up he marches her deeper into the forest hardly saying a word. They come to an isolated house which turns out to be his. She hears a snatch of conversation between men who are digging a grave by lantern-light. She runs away and is mad by the time she reaches home.

Nell's madness means that she is not able to tell anyone what has happened (making it difficult for a newspaper to report the story?). This sets up the possibility, and it is the openness of the poem that is its strength as elsewhere with Clare, that lurking in the forest is a serial killer who has struck before and will do so again. Ben is a shadowy, silent character who is not supplied with any rational motive. Perhaps however the whole story is in fact taking place inside Nell's head: Ben and the gravediggers are projections of her fears about masculinity. More real or in her head, this is still a Gothic nightmare. The forest is described as a dungeon and deep in its heart is an open grave with a spade lying by it: the poem is overflowing with sexual imagery. Does Ben subject his victims to that most Gothic of deaths, burial alive, or does he kill them first? Does he have sex with them before, or after, he has killed them? The role of the gravediggers is left chillingly unclear. To adapt Wilde, such a murder should be solitary and needed no accomplices (there are no accomplices to the murder in the forest that is described in 'March' in *The Shepherd's Calendar*). Perhaps the poem, told largely from Nell's point of view, is burying in its own grave what actually happened in the forest because it is so unspeakable. Her experience is a disturbing one, but is it bad enough to drive her crazy? Below the surface, in the grave, there is another poem lurking in which all manner of Gothic violence is possible. The world of the poem is dark, cruel and without any real explanation. Much of the imagery is explicitly sexual.

Radstock was aided and abetted in his crusade to clean up Clare's act by Eliza Emmerson. He also employed another go-between called Captain Sherwill who lectured Clare on gratitude. Emmerson was about ten years older than Clare and, unlike the Admiral, had literary pretensions, publishing poetry in newspapers and magazines. Her relationship with Clare was a very flirtatious one particularly early on, along some of the lines that the governess at Holywell had tried to establish. As has been seen, peasant-poets provoked sexualised responses which would not have been possible or legitimate in other circumstances. Clare allowed Emmerson to play to the full the parts of patroness and hostess even though she was not in the same league as the great hostesses of this period such as, say, Lady Holland. She nevertheless could affect to be with her very own peasant-poet as captive audience. She would probably have much preferred to have patronised Byron, but he was not available to her. Clare, far from being naïve, was usually a very acute and shrewd at reading people as proved yet again by the description of Emmerson in his autobiography:

> she has been a very pretty woman and is not amiss still and a womans pretty face is often very dangerous to her common sense for the notice she recievd in her young days threw an affectatious [air] about her feelings which she has not got shut of yet for she fancys that her friends are admirers of her person as a matter of course and

> acts accordingly which appears in the eyes of a stranger ridiculous enough but the grotesque wears off on becoming acquanted with better qu[a]litys and better qualitys she certanly has to counterballance them … (*BH*, p. 137)

Although there are breaks in their correspondence, Emmerson became Clare's most prolific correspondent. Most of his letters to her have not survived, which may or may not tell a story (it is some of the drafts that have survived). He mentions writing to her at one point requesting a portrait and confesses, more generally, to falling under her flirtatious spell. He acknowledges that at one time he thought that she was 'every thing' (*LJC*, p. 373). Emmerson bombarded him with advice and more occasionally with presents, which included cast-off clothes for his children and his wife. She sent six teaspoons and some sugar tongs engraved with her pen-name of Emma. She enjoyed playing the part of Lady Bountiful. She and Radstock became godparents by proxy in 1822 to Clare's daughter, Eliza Louisa, who was named after her. She was a bit of tease, a bit of a diva, a bit of a vamp. Younger poets were not entirely safe when she was around. Her relationships had to contain an element of intrigue, as Clare noticed (*LJC*, p. 351). She wrote not once but three times to Clare's wife while he was visiting London in 1824. The reports about his health were accompanied by a request to send the portrait of her, which he appears to have hidden away as instructed, up to London so that it could be framed and then hung up at Helpston.[57] She and her husband tried to help Clare sort out his finances after Taylor had given up publishing poetry. She was supportive when he undertook a traumatic move, or flitting, from Helpston to Northborough in 1832. With a theatrical flourish she sent money to buy a cow. She fantasised as always about doing a little light work alongside Clare in the garden: like Austen's Mrs Elton her version of pastoral was a very *cottage ornée* one.

Emmerson also played an important part in the editing and publication of Clare's final volume *The Rural Muse*. She chose the title, feeling that *The Midsummer Cushion* required too much explanation, and marked up the manuscript to indicate which poems were her 'favourites'.[58] She probably altered the titles of some individual poems. One of the publishers, Jeremiah How, took her advice. Probably prompted by her, he also made a successful application on Clare's behalf to the Royal Literary Fund which gave him fifty pounds. It is possible to see this sequence of events in the 1830s – the move to Northborough, the publication of the fourth volume and the Literary

Fund grant – as stabilising not just Clare's finances but his literary life more generally. Yet it is probably more accurate to say that the damage had already been done. If he had been able to move to a smallholding that offered the prospect of self-sufficiency in the earlier 1820s, then his literary life might have been a very different story. If Radstock had not taken him up as an Evangelical as opposed to a literary crusade, then things might have been different as well.

The relationship between the poet and Eliza Emmerson, this highly theatrical admirer (every bit as camp in her way as Wainewright and the Londoners), certainly stood the test of time. It began, however, with her acting as a go-between for Radstock, explaining his paternal feeling for Clare and trying to make sure that the poet played the part of a dutiful and grateful son. She often played the good cop to Radstock's bad cop. Radstock had several sons, so it is not quite clear why he wanted to adopt another. Eliza became involved in Radstock's attempt to get what he considered to be those very incriminating letters back from Clare: 'the world are not sufficiently liberal to understand the nature of such friendships'.[59] She passed on the Admiral's reasons for wanting to get rid of the offending passage about wealth: 'tell Clare if he has still a recollection of what I have done, and am still doing for him, he must give me unquestionable *proofs*, of being that man I would have him to be –'.[60] Taylor noted that Radstock had a voracious appetite for flattery and, it could be added, for getting his own way. Clare had 'to act the puppet while he pulls the strings'.[61] Radstock, like some of the Londoners, had to be the centre of attention despite his attempts to dress up his actions in a more self-effacing religious rhetoric. He was never entirely convinced about Clare's political correctness, despite the removal of this passage. He detected more radicalism in 'The Village Minstrel', writing 'This is radical slang' against two stanzas, and warned the poet to steer well clear of satire.[62] Clare may have initially responded favourably to the Admiral's straightforward manner with its appearance of common sense and appreciated the efforts that were made on his behalf. There is also enough evidence to suggest that, after a relatively brief honeymoon period, he felt some irritation at the high-handed actions of this bullying busybody from the Vice Society. Emmerson in her role as good cop often praised some of Clare's more explicitly political poetry, while warning him against publishing it.[63]

Emmerson's letters to Clare are often over-the-top and rather silly. She was an exhausting penpal (and modern readers do not, of course, have to reply to her). She gave some good advice, for instance about his increasing preoccupation with Elizabethan poetry, but this was mixed with attempts to get him to deal more conventionally with nature and sensibility. Some of the letters were short, but most of them were what she described as 'long chit chat' ones.[64] She nevertheless developed into a loyal friend and supporter. It appears that some of Clare's letters to her may have been frank and confessional. There is some discussion in 1826 of an 'outbreaking from propriety', which probably meant that he had told her about a relationship with a local woman (perhaps he was also a bit of a tease occasionally).[65] There had been an earlier confession as well. Emmerson and her husband made a point of visiting him in 1825, staying at an inn in nearby Market Deeping. One of the reasons they may have visited was perhaps to try to retrieve Radstock's illegible letters. Eliza was also worried, as she had some cause to be, about the content of some of her own letters to Clare. She was enough of a prima donna, however, to want to picture him re-reading them until his death. They could be returned then, she tells him. All this Gothic paranoia about letters suggests that not all the biographical evidence is currently available, but since letters have been destroyed it may never be.

The mid-1820s represented a watershed in Clare's literary life. His connections with the *London Magazine* came to an end. The publication of *The Shepherd's Calendar* continued to be delayed and Taylor was in the process of winding up the firm that had first brought him to the attention of the reading public. A number of projects, for instance his autobiography, had been started and then not brought to fruition in terms of publication. Radstock at times had tried to boss him about as if he were a potentially mutinous sailor from the lower decks and yet his death was probably still a blow. Gilchrist had died two years before in 1823, depriving Clare of his chief source of literary gossip and support in the locality. Bloomfield's death in the same year was another blow (even though Clare had been too drunk to visit him on his way back from London in 1822). Clare's isolation should still not be exaggerated: he maintained contacts with Stamford as well as with some of the upper-servants at Milton Hall such as Edmund Artis and Joseph Henderson, who were both very educated people.[66] Writing, except for the stage and journalistic page, was almost by definition an isolated and isolating activity for some of the time. Isolation can also be a loaded term carrying a lot of class assumptions: Lockhart and his kind expected shop assistants (Keats), governesses (Charlotte and Anne Brontë) and peasants (Clare) to lead isolated lives. Charlotte Brontë may have moaned about Haworth being an obscure hill village but, for its size, it had a rich cultural life. There were times when Clare described Helpston as being the back-of-beyond: 'I live here among the ignorant like a lost man' (*LJC*, p. 230). Yet being close to Stamford meant in turn being close to a thriving centre of provincial culture. It is necessary, despite what restless writers may sometimes say themselves, not to get drawn unwittingly into reproducing snobbish assumptions that culture can only exist amongst an educated elite in places like Edinburgh and London.

Clare's dream of becoming a professional writer, which was still just a possibility in 1825, was fading fast. He clung tenaciously to it (some critics praise the maturity of his work in the late 1820s and earlier 1830s, but increasingly in face of the evidence). He visited London again in 1828 for about five weeks, and yet his identity was now that of an invalid rather than a literary lion. He took sulphur baths and some acquaintances wrote to complain that he had not visited them. Bloomfield had advised him to 'let nothing prevent you from writing'.[67] This is just what he did, and what in turn gives his literary life its uplifting qualities. Although he would come to be constructed as a result of his alleged madness as a pathetic figure deserving sympathy, this denies his resolve. He was not allowed to become a professional writer as this identity was not in the script, and yet his output exceeded most of those who were professionals. He was a victim in some respects, but not in others.[68] He had good days and bad days, yet carried on writing almost to the very end. This is why, even though he has been critically unfashionable until relatively recently, he has usually been admired by other writers, particularly poets, as shown here in some of the endnotes. He is a writer's writer. He scribbled away in the fields, while his children were noising around him (as he put it) and in the bleak world of the asylums after a short break when he first got there. Nothing could, or did, stop him for long. Readers eventually came and then, just as abruptly and mysteriously, went, but he still carried on writing away. In adversity I struggled on: there is a joy in writing no matter what the daily cares might be, to paraphrase him. As noted, joy is indeed a word that reverberates throughout his poetry: the finding of it through poetry, the losing of it and the attempts to recover it.

While Radstock was recovering from his fall he still managed to write to Herbert Marsh, the Bishop of Peterborough, to get him to support his local poet. Marsh, who was also a Professor at Cambridge, was renowned for his strong and often controversial views, particularly about the way in which dissenters were trying to infiltrate the state church and undermine it, or level it, from within. He made anyone seeking either a living or curacy within his diocese answer a whole series of questions, 87 in all, designed to flush out the merest suspicion of support for dissent. This practice landed him in a certain amount of hot water: he twice had to speak against petitions that had been presented to the House of Lords questioning the use of these questions.[69] Clare, it will be remembered, had some sympathies with dissent and so may not have been entirely at ease in the presence of this very high churchman. Having said this, he seems to have appreciated Marsh's gifts and visits. Marsh was one of a number of people who furthered his interest in the Renaissance, giving him a copy of a memoir of Queen Elizabeth's court. Although he did occasionally draft independent letters to some of his patrons, he was for the most part surprisingly diplomatic. He was patronised by staunch Tories such as Radstock and Marsh, as well as by Whigs such as the Fitzwilliams. Between these extremes there were the civic reformers, and also the wits and wags from the *London Magazine*. There were quarrels, for instance with Radstock and Drury, but what is perhaps more remarkable is that Clare generally speaking won and maintained the respect of these very different interest groups. He was not being merely rhetorical when he claimed to have friends on different political sides.

Clare formed a closer relationship with Marsh's German wife, Marianne, than he did with the formidable bishop himself. She appears to have been kindly and attentive: giving him a silver coronation medal, medicine, plants for the garden and presents for the children. She also sent books for him and his children, as well as a magnifying glass to help with his botanical studies. One of the books was on epitaphs. As indicated earlier, Clare had something of an obsession with tombstones. Marsh's female companion gave him a steel-nibbed pen. It seems that he also made, or tried to make, gifts, when he was able to, writing to Taylor to ask for some of Keats's poems to give to one of Marsh's sons (*LJC*, p. 480). Although this relationship began in 1820 (Marianne Marsh paid at least two visits in this year), it seems to have become particularly important towards the end of the decade after Clare had lost as has been seen many of his earlier friends and supporters. The Bishop and his wife were however often away from Peterborough, spending nearly six months at Hastings for instance in 1828–9. When Clare was well enough, he spent time at the Bishop's Palace. At other times his wife went over to collect medicines. Both Radstock and Emmerson in their different ways wanted to hear that squawk of flattery: admire my endless, fatherly efforts on your behalf, my son; admire me as a woman because everybody else, and I mean everybody darling, has done. This is not the case with Marianne Marsh, who addresses Clare with quiet dignity as 'My Dear Mr. Clare'. He writes back to 'My dear Madam' (*LJC*, p. 543). Emmerson, by contrast, was not nearly so restrained in the letters that she wrote to 'My very dear Clare', who is also more occasionally called 'Johnny'. Clare writes back to 'My dear Eliza' (*LJC*, p. 460). He feels at ease in his letters to Marsh, as he sometimes is in ones to Taylor (*LJC*, pp. 499–501), to explore political issues openly and tentatively without fear of counter-revolutionary reprisals. He apologises for not returning a book by noting the dangers of walking around the countryside during the Swing Agricultural Riots of 1830/1: 'I fear there is even in our day a class of desperadoes little or no better than the rabble that made up the army of Jack Cade' (*LJC*, p. 543). He is making a literary reference to Shakespeare's *2 Henry VI*. The question of parliamentary reform makes him wonder whether there could be a common sense rather than party solution: 'for common sense is the right use of reason among common people who have no advantages of education to come at by different ways' (*LJC*, p. 556). This letter also has some commentary on Cobbett. Clare has time for him as a grammarian (the only one for whom he had any time), but not as a politician. He hopes that the mob on the one hand and party political 'spouters' on the other will not prevent 'a reform that would do good & hurt none' (*LJC*, p. 560). Once again, he is taking up positions that are close to those advanced by John Scott. The Marshes did their bit in helping to raise subscriptions for the fourth volume and kept in some sort of touch with his wife after he was taken to the asylum.[70]

Talking of spouting, Clare attended a performance of *The Merchant of Venice* in Peterborough in 1830 with the Bishop and his wife. He apparently ranted and raved at Shylock, and then made his own exit from the theatre. Some biographies suggest that this event foreshadows the madness that eventually engulfed him.[71] The move to Northborough in 1832 is then often seen as another significant milestone on the road to the asylums. Yet it was quite common in this period for spectators to heckle actors and indeed each other. Regency theatres were often very noisy places. The actress Fanny Kelly was shot at by a spectator who apparently objected to the way in which she often dressed up as a man. Byron and his chums kicked up a row one night at the Haymarket Theatre just after they had left school. Queen Caroline descended on the theatres to try to whip up support for her cause. Edmund Kean made his London debut as Shylock, winning noisy and sympathetic approval for the character. Although the theatre was half-empty, he still caused a sensation not least because he wore a black wig rather than the traditional red one.[72] Hazlitt reviewed the performance for the *Morning Chronicle*. Clare was taken to see Kean in 1820. Austen had been taken to see him in 1814, shortly after this début performance as Shylock. As will become clearer, it is by no means certain that Clare was clinically mad and therefore dangerous to go in search of earlier manifestations of his condition. Although not stated quite as explicitly as this, biographies tend to give the impression of him as an unsophisticated member of the audience who was not able to distinguish between illusion and reality. This then becomes the evidence for the delusions of madness. Yet Clare had attended the London theatres, which many others in the audience had probably not done. He had probably read more Renaissance drama than anybody else there, the actors included. Far from being a country bumpkin who did not know how to behave, perhaps he was just showing people in Peterborough how things were done in London. The event does not appear to have harmed his relationship with Marianne Marsh who, in a low-key way perhaps, represents many of the virtues and few of the vices of literary philanthropy. One of his local friends heard about the 'unfortunate affair at the Theatre at Peterboro' and urged him to apologise as quickly as possible.[73] His apology was graciously accepted.

Good Old Chuckey

Before being theatrically discovered as a Regency peasant-poet, Clare had relied quite heavily on his parents' opinions about his writings. He nevertheless adopted cover stories that concealed his authorship from them: asking them for opinions on poems and ballads as if he was collecting them rather than actually writing them himself. Clare's independent and ambitious streak was perhaps inevitably at odds with other feelings of dependence and insecurity. It is difficult to say just how literate his parents were in the conventional sense: probably not very. There is less doubt however that they, perhaps particularly his father, were extremely literate in, and knowledgeable about, folk traditions: the literacy of ear and memory. The mother in *The Shepherd's Calendar* is associated with story-telling.

Taylor has received a bad press from some critics and editors, who hold him largely responsible for damaging what is held to be distinctive about Clare's work. Yet, looked at historically, without Taylor there might not have been Clare and his literary life. At the best the poet might have had his trifles published locally by a Henson, a Ridge or a Drury and then been quickly forgotten. It was his connection with Taylor and the *London Magazine* that brought him to prominence. Radstock would not have wasted his time crusading on behalf of a very obscure local poet. It was also this connection that made him in others ways. As indicated, his reading perhaps particularly of Renaissance works and therefore his writing were influenced by many of the *London Magazine*'s agendas. Although not possible to document here in any detail, his knowledge of Renaissance writings was formidable.

Taylor was very much a hands-on editor which annoyed some of his authors such as Walter Savage Landor. He also saw part of his role as acting as a gatekeeper to make sure that poems, or parts of poems, that might be deemed to be offensive did not get published without revision. This was common practice at this time of acute social tension. It was the publisher rather than the author who was usually liable in prosecutions initiated by the Vice Society and others. Readers could also vote with their feet against a publishing house if they were offended by particular volumes. As mentioned, even a powerful patrician figure like Byron and his radical colleagues were worried about the consequences of offending the reading public. His publisher censored parts of the earlier cantos of *Don Juan*. Taylor's editing, by turns progressive treating a peasant-poet very seriously as a writer and by turns more cautious, needs to be set in this wider context.

Drury noted that Taylor made his selection for *Poems Descriptive* on the basis of trying to exclude material that might 'damn the book'.[74] As the row with Radstock indicates, Taylor took a broader view than some about what was acceptable. Clare, who was to confess later that his own judgement was very green at the beginning of his career, usually gives Taylor credit for improving his work. He acknowledged, mixing up his metaphors rather badly, that Taylor usually wielded his 'pruning hook' effectively because he knew 'what sort of a dish will suit the publics appetite better then I' (*LJC*, p. 204). In general terms, this was Clare's attitude throughout much of the time that he was being published by Taylor. He claimed that he himself could only distinguish between the good and bad parts of a poem when it was in print. He saw Taylor as providing a protective screen between him and the reading public. He was, as mentioned, both extremely shy and extremely ambitious: Taylor tried to conquer the latter and facilitate the former. It is not a bad thing to have done.

Clare's working relationship with Taylor was good. They had their pet names for each other: good old Chuckey and Johnny. What is not always brought out in some accounts of this relationship is just how demanding Clare could be. He liked and needed to have his ego massaged regularly, as many writers do. He was very, very boring and selfish about his real and imaginary illnesses: whining and whingeing, moaning and groaning. Taylor had to put up with threats of suicide, respond with advice on making a will and run errands for Clare, such as getting him a new seal. He also put the poet in touch with one of the doctors who had attended Keats, as well as John Scott. Perhaps all this was just a bit beyond the call of duty for a publisher, who had many other commitments. Clare expected Taylor to revise, or mend, his work and so could be slapdash, or what Taylor referred to as slovenly, with his drafts. Revising was not his strong suit early on in his career. Taylor often complained about Clare's handwriting.

Although there were some ups and downs, things did not really start to go seriously wrong with the relationship until the beginning of 1823. Taylor's father died in this year. Taylor, busy editing the *London Magazine* as well as trying to rescue his failing business, did not have the same amount of time to spare Clare. He describes himself as leading the exhausting life of 'bookseller, publisher, editor, author & printer's devil to the London Magazine'.[75] Later on Taylor, a workaholic and something of a control freak, seems to have had a serious illness. His partner Hessey writes to Clare in September 1825 with an account of how physical symptoms eventually produced 'a high state of delirium'.[76] Clare himself had been ill throughout much of 1824. Perhaps it should come as no real surprise that these two walking wounded took such a long time to get a book out. There were faults on both sides as with any relationship: Taylor lost parts of *The Shepherd's Calendar* and, more generally, appears to have lost interest in the project. In addition to finding it hard to delegate, Taylor could also be indecisive (he never got around to producing his own biographies or editions of Keats and Clare despite being uniquely placed to do so). Clare wrote to him in 1825 asking if he wanted to abandon *The Shepherd's Calendar* project (*LJC*, p. 330). It was yet another lovers' tiff. A 'paper war' (*LJC*, p. 361) began. Taylor was obviously fond of Clare, if also sometimes exasperated by him, in much the same way as he might have been by a black-sheep brother. In addition to playing the part of a peasant-poet, Clare had to juggle with a number of other identities: dutiful son (Radstock), admiring toy boy (Emmerson) and, perhaps, as some sort of brother/buddy with Taylor. Taylor seems to have led something of a double life. He surrounded himself with drunks, addicts and womanisers, and yet also managed to distance himself from this world and take the high moral ground. He could, as Clare notes, be aloof and inscrutable. Yet there were also occasions such as the *London Magazine* dinners when he could be more unbuttoned. He could be moralistic one moment, and very camp the next. The appointment of a sub-editor to work on the poem, who was then not properly briefed and had problems of his own, did not help matters. If ever a book was jinxed, it was this one. There were even last-minute delays over the frontispiece. Perhaps they should have asked Wainewright to do it after all. Clare's run of bad luck continued. His fourth volume was delayed by the deaths of not one, but two partners, in the new firm that the Emmersons and others had worked hard to find for him. Perhaps it was not just bad luck, but an inability (for understandable reasons) to play the literary game.

The partisan nature of some Clare criticism means that much is made of Taylor's faults. He is not given enough credit for being at the progressive end of Regency publishing at a time when many others were walking the tightrope about what could and could not be said in print. By the same token, not enough is said about how extremely difficult to work with Clare could be at times. Or, at a more practical level, that there were inevitably communication problems between London and Helpston. Writers do not have to be made into boring pictures of perfection in order for them and their literary lives to excite the interest and enthusiasm that they deserve. Clare criticism needs to resist being pushed by some modern editors down the blind alley of having to take sides over Taylor's editorial policies. This is not being historical. The poems were edited according to the conventions of the day by a progressive publishing house that was prepared to take Clare very seriously as a writer. It is difficult to think of another house at this time that would have been prepared to have invested so much time and effort in him, as opposed to just publishing him as a one-off curiosity. It took him a long time to find another publisher and most of the smaller publishing ventures that he attempted independently of Taylor were not successful. Taylor helped Emmerson edit *The Rural Muse*, even though he had given up publishing poetry for some time.[77]

One of the legacies of Romanticism is a model of literary lives in which solitary, and often alienated, male geniuses labour to create works that are uniquely and distinctively their own. These works then become contaminated when they come into contact with the literary marketplace, which is seen as existing in a separate sphere. This is the view that seems to underpin the recent Clarendon editions of Clare: the authentic text is always the author's text before it reaches the marketplace. The terminology is fraught with problems. Perhaps there are just different texts, all of interest, rather than one sacred object. Even if the terms are accepted, it seems unlikely with such a prolific writer as Clare that the unedited text is always the one to be preferred. This is a model in which the text as property belongs exclusively to the individual author. Clare, a great imitator of Renaissance and eighteenth-century writings, might be somewhat amused as well as bemused by this. He was also at times, as mentioned, a self-conscious literary forger in the manner of Chatterton. Alternative models place much more emphasis on different forms of collaboration. The text, far from being unique and sacred, is an act of collaboration between an author and other writers. Perhaps all texts consist of borrowings, reworkings and rewritings. There are other models in which readers are allowed to become much more active and creative, each one producing different meanings from the same text and thus establishing their particular ownership of it. It is not necessary to take off into the higher realms of literary theory to wonder exactly what, if anything, is actually meant by authenticity. As far as Taylor's role is concerned, a model that suggests that authors and publishers are collaborators existing in the same sphere rather than inevitably being antagonists seems to be appropriate. They work together, more often than not in harmony, to create a text in accordance with the material and cultural conditions for production at a particular historical moment. They may transgress certain conventions, but they are still part of an historically determined process. This process is determined but not rigid, continually evolving and changing as a result of a complex series of cultural negotiations in which they, but also others such as readers, take part. Taylor and Clare were collaborators. They had differences of opinion, although the main reason that they fell out was that Taylor was too committed elsewhere to sustain such a demanding relationship, and Clare could be very demanding indeed, on a continuous basis.

Readers must of course make up their own minds about these editorial issues, as they are too complex to be dealt with at length here. Although dictionaries and others texts went some way towards standardising spelling during the eighteenth century, many writers from higher social backgrounds than Clare's retained their own eccentricities and peculiarities. There are some ingenious accounts that explain Austen's erratic spelling in terms of a self-conscious strategy to make sure that nobody would ever dream of letting her become a governess. Perhaps she was just not very good at spelling. The juvenilia produced by the Brontës into their late teens and beyond is riddled with spelling mistakes and contains little punctuation. Even though it may not have been intended for publication, the more general point is that Clare was not unique in producing manuscripts that needed some basic editing. A poem considered earlier, 'Crazy Nell', was however so heavily punctuated in its published version that its flow, and therefore sense, is in danger of getting lost, and this sort of thing happened quite a lot although not all the time.

Clare received a lot of useless advice about how and what to write at the start of his career. One of his correspondents nevertheless got close to identifying something that was important about his writing when he claimed that 'Yours is not that Panoramic view of Nature, which (imposing while viewed at a distance) only gives an idea of the general effect of the landscape: but you have touched your miniature with the finest pencil; every leaf and every flower is there accurately delineatd, & the minutia of nature's treasures revealed.'[78] This underestimates Clare's literariness: he is working in a tradition that goes back to Edmund Spenser's *The Shepheardes Calender* (1579) and beyond in his own *The Shepherd's Calendar*. It also overstates its own case as there is often a tension in the writing, as John Barrell and others have noticed, between the general and the particular. It nevertheless provides a reminder that those who produced selective panoramic descriptions in topographical poems needed to be looking down on the landscape rather than being a part of it. The panoramic view produced by an overseer (a far from neutral term as Clare himself indicates in 'The Parish') encoded ideas of social standing and ownership that were alien to his own experiences as a labourer, no matter how many times he encountered them in the pastoral poetry of the period. This is what produced the tension. Barrell notices in 'Hollywell', a poem that was considered earlier, that although Clare includes conventional descriptions of views and prospects he is much more at home with the 'immediate foreground'.[79] This is one of the reasons why he does not produce a conventional celebration of General Reynardson and his seat. Taylor and Hessey did not just perform the common and routine tasks for this period of correcting spelling, mending grammar and adding punctuation. As Clare usually submitted twice as much material as would fit into a standard-sized volume (determined by the price of paper), they and others urged him to become more of an overseer of the landscape as this would lead to more discrimination. Once again, this is a term loaded with ideological implications producing a chain of contradictions. Poets can discriminate, but can peasants?

Detail was often of crucial significance to Clare not just because it reflected his own particular position within as opposed to surveying the landscape, but also because his poetry increasingly became a refuge, almost a secretive hiding place despite its public nature, for a disappearing world. As suggested earlier, this impetus can be seen in an early poem like 'Hollywell' in which potential patrons have to be all but banished from the landscape in order for the poet to reclaim and celebrate it as his own. The poem as refuge is a theme that is developed even more passionately in *The Shepherd's Calendar*:

Old customs O I love the sound
However simple they may be
What ere wi time has sanction found
Is welcome & is dear to me
Pride grows above simplicity
& spurns it from her haughty mind
& soon the poets song will be
The only refuge they can find
(*MP*, 1, p. 158)

This comes from 'December' (the poem, as its title suggests, is like Spenser's organised around the months of the year) and, although Clare appears to be predicting this vital role in the near future for 'the poets song', the implication of much of the rest of the poem is that it has already arrived. He takes refuge in the past in *The Shepherd's Calendar*, while at the same time providing a refuge for memories of the past, including the opportunities for leisure that were available to labourers. This is also a main theme in poems like 'St Martins Eve'. Clare's calendar is like a time-capsule: it has to be packed and crammed with detail because no other record may be left. Taylor certainly tried to get Clare to resist this tendency, arguing in favour of selection and against a 'complete record of country affairs'.[80] Clare gives in 'May' in the unedited version a very long catalogue of wild flowers, 'My wild field catalogue of flowers' (*MP*, 1, p. 65), as he believes that those that have not already disappeared will soon be blighted out of existence. Mildew will be everywhere. Readers may find this catalogue 'Tedious and long' (*MP*, 1, p. 65), but the poet himself insists that this kind of detail is essential. This month also contains a catalogue of birds. There are plenty of other individual examples of this cataloguing tendency. The poem as a whole can also be seen as a catalogue. Every detail, or seeming trifle, needs to be treated reverently and with respect as a relic, perhaps the only one that might be left in a few years' time, from a rural world of childhood innocence that has been lost thanks to pride and some of its specific manifestations such as enclosure. The poem becomes an act of remembrance and of record. The poet is somebody for whom 'every trifle will his eye detain' (*MP*, 1, p. 137). As Clare might have been patronisingly introduced to the reading public by Henson as a writer of mere trifles, he reappropriates the term and invests it with significance and importance. And he remains true to his particular sense of the importance of the seemingly trivial. He maintains in an asylum poem called 'The Peasant Poet' that 'every thing' is worthy of being 'surveyed' by the poet's eye right down to the smallest insects (*LP*, 2, p. 845).

Clare is not a dialect poet but, rather, one who is not afraid to use dialect words and expressions to improve the sound of a poem. As mentioned, John Lucas (himself a poet as well as a critic) is quite right to insist that the poems need to be read with the ear as well as with the eye. Taylor added a glossary to *Poems Descriptive* in which some of the dialect words used are translated and had more sympathy with Clare's experiments with language than is sometimes claimed to be the case, at least early on in Clare's career. Having said this, he still removed dialect particularly if he felt that it would not be easily understood outside of Clare's immediate locality. And this obviously represented something of a Catch-22 situation, since dialect and district are by definition intimately connected. Johanna Clare nevertheless suggests that Clare's language, the language of the rural working class, might not just have been confined to one particular place.[81] There is some truth in this: Clare spent time working in Newark, and the militia that he was a member of had a reasonably large catchment area. He does not appear to have had any problems making himself understood when he escaped from the asylum in Essex and tramped back towards his home.

One of Clare's great strengths is the way he coins or mints his own language, sometimes using dialect and sometimes not, to suit particular occasions. For example in 'March' his language conveys a sense of struggle as the agricultural community wearily tries to get back to something like normal after the dead months of winter:

> The ploughman mawls along the doughy sloughs
> & often stop their songs to clean their ploughs
> From teazing twitch that in the spongy soil
> Clings round the colter terrfying toil
> The sower striding oer his dirty way
> Sinks anckle deep in pudgy sloughs & clay

> & oer his heavy hopper stoutly leans
> Strewing wi swinging arms the pattering beans
> (*MP*, 1, p. 40)

There are a couple of dialect words here: 'mawls' and (perhaps) 'colter'. Yet the passage does not depend on them but rather on literary devices such as rhyme, alliteration and onomatopoeia ('doughy', 'spongy', 'pudgy' and so on). Earlier on in 1821 Clare tried to draw a distinction between dialect and what he described as a more universal 'expressive' (*LJC*, p. 168) vocabulary. It is this 'expressive' vocabulary that is one of the great strengths of *The Shepherd's Calendar*, and of his poetry more generally.[82] All language is, or is meant to be, 'expressive' in a general sense. What Clare appears to mean here, however, is that he is concerned to arrest the reader's attention by using unusual, but still understandable, words and phrases. The poems become a refuge not just for old customs, but also for a vocabulary that requires preservation. This is not however a rigidly antiquarian exercise because, as implied, Clare is actively playing with words, and their expressive sounds and possible meanings, and encouraging his readers to do the same. It is only possible here to hint at the richness of this vocabulary: chelping (gossiping), flitting (moving house), jobbling (swaying), moozing (dozing), proggling (poking), sluttering (sliding) and toltering (hobbling). Readers can, and should, compile their own lists, or consult the ones usefully provided by the Clarendon editors. It will be seen in the next chapter that Dickens adopted a very dismissive attitude towards Clare. This disguises the fact that they both played with language and its plurality in order to challenge the monologic discourses of their time.

The Clarendon editions show which poems were not deemed fit for publication during Clare's literary life, and how those that were had had the pruning hook taken to them (often though with Clare's consent). And increasing amounts of his prose writings are now becoming easily available for the first time. As some of his manuscripts are very difficult indeed to decipher and sequence, these various editions clearly represent scholarly landmarks. As far as his literary life is concerned, the important point is to use such editions not to get drawn down blind alleys where the debate is a somewhat old-fashioned one about authors and their authenticity but, rather, to get a sense of just what was available to Victorian and later readers and what was not. In other words, the editions need to be incorporated into arguments about reception. Clare's marginality has been caused by big issues such as class prejudice. It has also been caused at a more specific level by the unavailability of writings that might have interested these later readers more than the ones that were actually in print in the form that they were. Such a view will be explored in the next chapter. Although this kind of argument has to be speculative, there is a case for saying that as far as Clare's reputation was concerned there were some missed opportunities in the early Victorian period. This does not mean, however, losing sight of the fact that Taylor was at the progressive end of Regency publishing. He may at times have been a bit prim and proper, yet it is still important to remember that as publisher it was his head rather than Clare's that would have been on the block if there had been very serious objections to the poetry. As Byron and his friends realised, the cultural climate of the early 1820s made the publication of poetry that might be seen as radical in both form and content a dangerous enterprise. Taylor remains however something of an enigma. He was capable of demanding correct grammar and morality, while at the same time editing a camp magazine and surrounding himself with some writers who liked to walk on the wild(e) side. What can be argued with much more certainty is that he took Clare very seriously indeed as a writer, at a time when Lockhart and many others were trashing and ridiculing writers whom they felt were not members of their elite literary club or coterie. The attacks were not just confined to the pages of the periodical press, as John Scott was to find to his cost out on that foggy duelling ground at Chalk Farm. Championing Cockneys and peasants at this time was not something to be undertaken at all lightly.

3
The Importance of Being Earnest: Manly Artisans and Sincere Sages

Our own daily realities

Taylor blamed the commercial failure of The *Shepherd's Calendar* on the fact that poetry was increasingly becoming a luxury item, and declared that readers now preferred works of utility.[1] Reverting to his more serious side, he went off to supply such works to the University of London. The Regency period was rapidly giving way to the early Victorian one. Thomas Carlyle's first publication was in the *London Magazine*, but he quickly distanced himself from this frivolous world. His social criticism came to define and then dominate Condition-of-England debates in the 1830s and 1840s. He exhorted the artisan-writers such as Thomas Cooper, Ebenezer Elliott and Samuel Bamford who were replacing peasant-poets like Clare to concentrate on factual prose that made realistic, topical and thus useful contributions to these debates.

Although Carlyle was not asked in advance, he was nevertheless reasonably flattered to have Cooper's epic poem, *The Purgatory of Suicides* (1845), dedicated to him. He was still at pains however to distance and detach himself from mere poetry more generally:

> I think that I would recommend you to try your next work in *Prose*, and as a thing turning altogether on Facts, not Fictions. Certainly the *music* that is very traceable here might serve to irradiate into harmony far profitabler things than what are commonly called "Poems", – for which, at any rate, the taste in these days seems to be irrevocably in abeyance. We have too horrible a practical chaos round us; out of which every man is called by the birth of him to make a bit of *COSMOS*: that seems to me to be the real poem for a man – especially at present.[2]

Carlyle, the sage or prophet who self-consciously cultivated Old Testament rhythms and cadences along with obscure Germanic sentences, and his disciples were searching for manly, robust artisan writers who could illuminate if not always answer the Condition-of-England question. Clare and his work, in the form in which it was available, were not seen as fitting this urgent and topical agenda.

A suspicion of poetry surfaces again and again during the period of Clare's increasing marginalisation, perhaps sometimes because it was not regarded as a truly manly activity. One of Carlyle's most dedicated disciples, J.H. Sterling (a clergyman), sneered at what he took to be the complete and utter irrelevance of Alfred Tennyson's poetry in *The Quarterly Review* in 1842, reiterating criticisms that had been made of Tennyson's earlier work, and indeed of Keats's poetry as well: 'The verse is full of liquid intoxications, and the language of golden oneness. While we read, we too are wandering, led by Nymphs, among the thousand isles of old mythology, and the present fades away from us into a pale vapour. To bewitch us with our own daily realities and not with their unreal opposites, is a still higher task...' (90, p. 401). This sturdy emphasis on 'our own daily realities' permeated many early Victorian periodicals. *Eliza Cook's Journal* declared in 1850, confirming Taylor's reading of the signs of the times, that 'the popular appetite is now for something real, life-like, and written with a purpose' (2, p. 219). It was not just explicitly social-problem journals that sang from this hymn sheet. *The Cambridge and Oxford Review* maintained in 1845 that the 'first requisite for poets' was 'sincerity' (1, p. 66). They were expected to tell something called the whole truth. One of Clare's earliest surviving letters, to Holland, declared that a concern for truth 'crampt' (*LJC*, p. 13) the imagination, even though as has been seen some of his early poems may have been initially based on stories from the newspapers.

Carlyle was the great scourge of Regency values, despite some of his own stylistic frivolities and masquerades, eccentric and self-conscious mannerisms. He was absolutely disgusted when he met Charles Lamb in 1831, sponging drinks and attempting to be frivolous about the serious in the manner of high Regency camp. He thought that this Regency relic was mad, and perhaps effeminate as well (although the cleaned-up, sobered-up, cosy version of Lamb did have his Victorian admirers). Carlyle, who did an awful lot of pronouncing, pronounced that Sidney Smith's Regency wit was coarse, which hardly gets it right. Regency figures like Wainewright, Reynolds and Egan would have shocked him even more. His strict, puritanical sense of work discipline was deeply offended by the frivolous world of Regency dandies and their valets, and the whole hollow culture of what he termed valetism. He made connections between dandyism for the few and drudgery for the many, and thus more generally between the worlds of the greedy and the needy, the tailored and the tailors. This meant that his earlier criticism appealed to progressive radicals and early socialists (Marx and Engels), as well as to conservatives such as the Young England group. Regency valets and flunkies, as well as those peddling quack political remedies, had to be replaced by strong soldiers, of industry and intellect, who would steadfastly fight the good fight against chaos and anarchy with all of their manly might. Brave hearts were required.

Carlyle's influential study of *Chartism* (1839) opens on a shared note of anxiety that the French Revolution could be re-enacted here: 'A feeling very generally exists that the condition and disposition of the working classes is a rather ominous matter at present; that something ought to be said, something ought to be done, in regard to it.'[3] Carlyle and others were deeply afraid, or affected to be, that Chartism might overthrow the established order of things, plunging everyone and everything into the abyss. Such a response was conditioned by the way in which working-class movements tended to be interpreted from above, from the balcony window by an overseer, solely in terms of their sudden, dramatic and violent manifestations. This view could only be sustained, however, by ignoring the self-help, moral rearmament traditions within Chartism. According however to Carlyle's prophetic or visionary perspective, the Chartists were animals and their petitions, despite what was actually being said there in a highly constitutional language, 'bellowings, inarticulate cries as of a dumb creature in rage and pain; to the ear of wisdom they are inarticulate prayers: "Guide me, govern me! I am mad and miserable and cannot guide myself!"'[4]

Carlyle names and shames two sets of people for being responsible for Chartism (a series of largely working-class protest movements in the 1830s and 1840s) and thus for the perilous and precarious state of the nation. He blames, first of all, the traditional ruling class for selfishly pursuing their own leisure and pleasure in the manner of Regency excess rather than discharging their paternal duties and responsibilities. Yet he is also scathing about the claims of the emerging class of political economists, utilitarians and statisticians, with their quick quack remedies, to look after the best interests of the people. When he suggests that something needs to be done to help the bellowing Chartist animal, violent but also frightened, he does not have in mind a series of factual, statistical investigations. These sometimes only produced paralysis, or donothingness to use his own term. The language of fact is presented as embodying specific perspectives and points of view. It does not by itself produce strong, good governance.

When Carlyle advised poets like Cooper to deal with facts he meant them to concentrate on what documentary film-makers came to call the blazing fact of the matter, rather than to accumulate mere dry-as-dust facts for facts' sake. He himself rejected forms of mechanical quantification such as statistics, which were rapidly gaining cultural authority during the 1830s (being used and sometimes abused by asylums and other institutions), to search ever so diligently for a strictly limited number of essential, or emblematic, facts that could establish points about the quality of life, or lack of it. Matters factual are by no means always matters essential: 'Statistic Inquiry, with its limited means, with its short vision and headlong extensive dogmatism, as yet too often throws not light, but error worse than darkness.'[5] Just one carefully chosen and interpreted fact can, for the sincere sage, reveal the true Condition-of-England. Carlyle introduces the Stockport parents in the first chapter of *Past and Present* (1843). They have killed their three children so that they could get some money from a burial society in order to buy food for themselves. Carlyle comments: 'such instances are like the highest mountain apex emerged into view; under which lies a whole mountain region and land, not yet emerged'.[6] This one instance, or what would be called nowadays a human interest story, dramatically illuminates the Condition-of-England, showing how it has become natural to behave unnaturally. This was a method of social analysis frequently employed by early Victorian journals such as *Punch* and *The Illustrated London News*, as well as in the poetry of conscience such as 'The Song of the Shirt' by Thomas Hood (who had helped to edit the *London Magazine* under Taylor and with whom Clare corresponded about possible publication in later journals).

The artisan-writer was regarded by Carlyle and his followers as somebody who could add a vital human, qualitative dimension to social questions. This was of little or no help to Clare. Agricultural labourers were no longer the flavour of the period. Writers who were associated with forms of aristocratic patronage were also regarded, unfairly in Clare's case, as being deeply implicated in and compromised by literary valetism and flunkydom. Mary Leman Gillies, in an article on 'The Influence of the Aristocracy in Literature' for *The People's Journal* on 7 February 1846, applauded the fact, as she saw it, that literature was free 'from a servile devotion to mere rank and wealth' (p. 84). Such a view was very common in early Victorian periodicals.

The publication and reception of *The Purgatory of Suicides* shows the signs of the times that were working against Clare. The poem, which was written while Cooper was serving a two-year prison sentence for his Chartist activities (part of the conversion narrative), was sent to a number of publishers, two of whom stated that poetry was a drug in the market. When the humble hero of Thomas Miller's *Godfrey Malvern* (1842) arrives in London after publishing one volume of poetry, he is told that 'poetry has become quite a drug in the market'.[7] Although a convenient and very clichéd response that had been trotted out throughout the eighteenth century to fob off writers seen as being undesirable, there was still some truth in this. When the Brontë sisters published their poetry, at their own expense, in 1846 they probably sold only two volumes within a year. The equation between poetry and drugs is part of a wider set of associations with forms of intoxication. Poets and their readers risked becoming addicts. Writers such as Dickens, Benjamin Disraeli and Douglas Jerrold looked more sympathetically at Cooper's poem before its publication. They were primarily concerned about his potential to comment on the 'daily realities' of working-class life. Cooper could also set a good example by continuing to distance himself as much as possible from the violent, bellowing physical-force Chartism. The poem was eventually published by Jeremiah How, who had been involved with Clare's fourth volume.

Reviewers constantly reminded Cooper of his true vocation, of what sort of man they would have him to be. *Douglas Jerrold's Shilling Magazine* believed that such a writer 'cannot but produce other, and we think, superior works; and it would be a benefit to all classes if he would give a Chartist epic, prose or verse, depicting the genuine lives and characteristics of the people' (3, p. 96). *The Eclectic Review*, although finding faults, was more charitable towards Cooper, claiming that he had already produced 'a genuine poem springing out of the spirit of the times, enabled as he is by his powers and his position to reflect the reality unencumbered with the prejudices of rank or party'. The strength of the poem was connected with the strength of the artisan-poet, who is described as 'all bone and sinew' (18, pp. 671–2). The body, or imagined body, of the poet influences criticism of the body of his work. This is a form of homo-eroticism that dares not speak its name. Although Cooper's success depended upon his ability to convince middle-class social reformers that he was indeed their man of the moment, he also built up a working-class following. The poem was praised in the Chartist press and one of Clare's correspondents, Thomas Inskip, who visited him during the asylum years and got some of his poetry published in newspapers, was a fan of it. He mentions the poem in letters to Clare.[8]

Cooper's next two publications disappointed most reviewers because they did not make obviously useful contributions to burning social debates. *Douglas Jerrold's Shilling Magazine* reminded him yet again of exactly what was expected from an artisan writer in this period, to boldly go where no writer had apparently been before:

> The true office of such men is to record new experiences, and reveal new conditions of humanity; and this we earnestly entreat him to devote himself to ... The poor (that is nine tenths of the population) have never yet been truly represented as regards their characteristics, opinions, or condition. We know as little of their real condition as of the tribes of Africa, perhaps less. Yet here is one of themselves, who has the power of utterance and speaks not of them ... (3, p. 190)

Cooper sent 'Eyewitness' reports on 'The Condition of the People of England' to *Douglas Jerrold's Weekly Newspaper*. It was felt that his poetry had value only if it gave utterance to what were seen as being genuine, sincere and truthful insights on contemporary working-class life and culture.

Charles Kingsley's essay on 'Burns and His School' in 1859 noted 'the existence of a great and fearful gulf between those who have, and those who have not, in thought as well as in purse, which must be, the former article at least, bridged over as soon as possible, if we are to remain a people much longer'.[9] He wrote to Cooper, making it clear that artisan-writers had a sacred duty and mission to help social engineers like himself build the necessary bridges: 'I want some one like yourself, intimately acquainted with the mind of the working classes, to give me an insight into their life and thoughts, as may enable me to concentrate my powers effectually to their service.'[10] The artisan-poet has to labour to produce a commodity, called knowledge, which can then be used, or consumed, by literary professionals.

Cooper's life, and to a lesser extent his work, were raided and reconstructed by Kingsley for his social-problem novel *Alton Locke: Tailor and Poet* (1850). Escapism is the main impetus behind Alton's initial pursuit of poetry. He is a Cockney poet (although not in quite the same suburban sense as Keats and others had been labelled as such by *Blackwood's*) who wants only to read and write about what lies beyond his very limited experience. He nevertheless encounters the abrasive Sandy Mackaye, a bookseller who is the mouthpiece for Carlyle's views. Mackaye warns him against reading aristocratic, and it might be added Regency, writers like Byron. The aspiring poet is taken on a walk through the streets of London to show him the true facts of life and make him change his mind.

There is nevertheless a conflict between the advice Alton receives here and the demands of his upper-class patrons. It has been suggested that Dean Winnstay might have been based on one of Clare's own patrons, Bishop Marsh.[11] This is possible, although what is more immediately apparent about *Alton Locke* (and indeed *Godfrey Malvern*) is the way in which Clare is conspicuous by his absence from a novel that not only deals extensively with working-class poets, but also has quite substantial sections set in the Fens. Even if there are very occasional traces of Clare's story present, the novel as a whole provides an example of the way it had become almost forgotten, a memory lost, as Clare was to say, in the early Victorian period. It is Burns rather than Clare who becomes and remains the representative of the struggle to combine literature and labour. The Dean wants Alton's poetry to be based, not on his own experience, but rather on the repetition of established poetic forms. He is pleased that the poems 'evince on the whole, a far greater acquaintance with English classic models, and with the laws of rhyme and melody, than could have been expected from a young man of your class'. He is also concerned, as was Radstock, to make sure that patronage produces a suitably deferential, grateful poet: 'Now, recollect; if it should be hereafter in our power to assist your prospects in life, you must give up, once and for all, the bitter tone against the higher classes, which I am sorry to see in your MSS.'[12] Alton allows some of the more explicitly political passages to be edited out of his *Songs of the Highways*. Clare's story is both absent and present.

The rest of the novel shows Alton trying to be true to himself, despite the way in which he is initially flattered by patronage. It is eventually Eleanor, who has the Carlylean mission 'to find a man of the people whom I could train to be poet of the people', who gets him to abandon violent, bellowing Chartism in favour of a Christian Socialist emphasis on brotherhood.[13] He must write about 'daily realities', but in such a way as to bring out the possibilities for social reconciliation rather than conflict: building bridges again.

Although Kingsley himself was acutely aware, in *Yeast* (1850) as well as in *Alton Locke* itself, of rural poverty, many other early Victorian social critics tended to assume that 'daily realities' must, almost by definition, be either urban or metropolitan ones. Robinson and Summerfield suggest that Clare was 'damned because he was a peasant at a time when the national imagination was being captured by the immensity of industrialism'.[14] This may be true in general terms, although it does not register the way in which the artisans who were replacing the peasants came to represent a mythologised set of craft values that could sometimes be in opposition to industrialisation itself. William Johnson Fox was a Unitarian minister who transformed *The Monthly Repository* in the early 1830s into one of the leading journals of social reform, as well as of the dissidence of dissent. He asserts there, in a long article on 'The Poor and Their Poetry' in 1832, that 'the genuine poverty of society does not live in the fields. Its horrors and its passions, in their sternest form, are city born. Let there be meadows and mountains, but there must also be streets, alleys, workshops, and jails, to complete the scenery of the poetry of poverty. By neglecting these, Bloomfield and Clare have lost the best subjects for their best powers…They are too merely pastoral' (6, pp. 193–4).[15] It was extremely difficult for Clare to stage a poetic comeback in the face of such impossible demands. Dickens adopted an even more dismissive tone later when he claimed that Clare was a fine example of the 'preposterous exaggeration of small claims'.[16] He had more time for Bloomfield, who could be reclaimed as a metropolitan artisan, rather than being seen as a mere farmer's boy.

The quest for a working-class poet who could comment directly and explicitly on the Condition-of-England led Fox, Carlyle, Samuel Smiles and others to sing the praises of Ebenezer Elliott. *The New Monthly Magazine* confidently heralds the dawning of a new age in 1831 (when, it will be remembered, Clare was struggling to get his fourth volume into print):

> There is a tide in the affairs of poets as well as of other people, and that the author of the *Corn Law Rhymes* may make the best of that which is now setting in to his advantage, must be the wish of every one to whom genuine poetry is dear, accompanied, as in the present instance it is, by ornaments which poets are sometimes wont to neglect – genuine utility, and simple undisguised truth…Poetry, in the present case, is the handmaid of reality, and points to evils not drawn from the fruitful matrix of imagination, but existing in stern and withering permanence, as a national plague and a national dishonour. (33, pp. 444–5)

Such attempts to claim Elliott as the rough-hewn shape of things to come often missed the point that he was a prolific writer on rural life, or what he called 'ruralities'.[17] Fox turned a blind eye to this when he presented Elliott in *The Monthly Repository* as a working artisan whose life, very crudely and simply, informed his poetry (his class position was in fact more ambiguous than suggested here and elsewhere): 'His mind is healthy and vigorous; always knows its work; and the prominent passages are such as the subject naturally throws out, not such as are elaborated and polished with infinite pains for the production of effect' (6, p. 196). Effect, it is implied, is something which only appeals to the effete. Carlyle was also impressed by Elliott as 'an earnest truth-speaking man'. He differentiates this poet, with his 'rugged substantial English', as sharply as possible from the kind of writers who had attracted the condescending attention of Southey. Dropping into his back-to-front style, he pronounced: 'here too be it premised that nowise under the category of "uneducated poets", or in any fashion of dilettante patronage, can our Sheffield friend be produced'.[18] Elliott had in fact received advice and help from Southey, even though he was not included in the essay on the uneducated poets. Like Cooper, Elliott also had a following amongst the working classes themselves. Here again it was his perceived ability to speak something called the truth that was important. *The Poor Man's Guardian*, perhaps the most influential publication of the pauper press, comments on one of his poems: 'The painful picture which the author of "Corn-law Rhymes" has here painted is "taken from life". Those who are acquainted with the state of our manufacturing towns will readily recognise its truth' (79, 8 September 1832). Elliott himself defined poetry as 'sincerity in earnest'.[19]

Clare almost certainly became tainted by his association with dilettante patronage, even though as has been seen he was carefully and conveniently ignored by Southey. His poetry was held to be at best marginal, and at worst irrelevant, to what were taken to be 'daily realities'. He was not, however, completely neglected. *Eliza Cook's Journal* carried an article in 1851 which relates him to the education question: 'The life of Clare presents a striking and affecting example of the pursuit of knowledge under difficulties, but it also furnishes an exceeding painful illustration of the misery which is sometimes produced by the gift of poetry descending on a mind struggling in a humble station and without the requisite means of development and sustenance.' Referring to Clare's limited formal education, the article hopes that 'another generation will not be allowed to grow up to manhood without at least such provision being made for their education as to put the children of even the poorest classes in possession of the common rudiments of knowledge'. Clare's life provides useful ammunition for an argument about the Condition-of-England and yet it still has to be said that it was not used very often at all in this context. The article, entitled 'John Clare, The Northamptonshire Peasant', certainly promotes Clare while at the same time revealing the extent of his neglect and marginalisation. It is, for instance, riddled with factual errors as well as more conceptual ones. Clare is presented as a naïve, primitive writer who 'owed little to books, but wrote from the heart'.[20] His associations with the *London Magazine* and its agendas are neglected. Some of the occasional references to Clare in the journalism of this period are also more often than not based on misunderstandings about his life. A letter to *The Manchester Courier*, primarily concerned to champion the causes of local artisan writers such as J.C. Prince, suggests on 4 September 1846 that Clare was 'taken from the plough and put in possession of a farm', which is wrong on both counts. Clare had indeed been employed to 'drive plough' (*AW*, p. 54), but early on in his life as a labourer long before his theatrical discovery. His identity has become confused, and not for the first time, with that of a heaven-taught ploughman called Burns. The move to Northborough did not involve moving to rent-free accommodation, as he was at pains to point out when some periodicals got the story wrong.

The new breed of earnest patrons wanted to find poets in their own image. They also, like Southey, took some care to discover writers who did not threaten their own position as professional men of letters. Dickens was to dismiss Clare and yet spent time helping a London artisan of very limited ability, John Overs, to publish *Evenings of a Working Man, Being the Occupation of His Scanty Leisure* (1844). As noticed earlier, titles are texts in their own right. The full one here contains Dickens's own name. He wrote the Preface, or patron's text, in which he distances himself as sharply as possible from dilettante patronage. He claims (as indeed he has to) that Overs himself is not a neglected genius but, rather, an example of the potential within the working classes that might be realised through universal education. Some of the reviewers still chided Overs for revelling in historical romances rather than providing the necessary social commentary. *Tait's Edinburgh Magazine* spells out the name of the Condition-of-England game: 'It is now idle to speculate on how much better his stories might have been, if, instead of wandering through the regions of historical romance, he had, like his generous patron, Mr Dickens, confined his studies to the daily life in which he was an actor and observer' (11, p. 743). Once again, an allegedly idle literary wanderer, or soodler, is sternly advised to stick to the straight and narrow path. Dickens tried to use Overs as a source of information about working-class life, asking him for a response to Carlyle's *Chartism*. Here and on other occasions Overs did not always tell Dickens what he wanted to hear. Although there were certainly some important differences between old-style dilettante and philanthropic patronage and the newer patterns of patronage employed by Dickens, Kingsley and other Condition-of-England writers, there were also some striking similarities. Dickens sounds uncannily like Radstock when he tells the independent Overs that his 'conduct has disappointed me, and has shown me that you are not the sort of man I took you for'.[21]

Dickens's own ambivalent class position (the shadow of the debtors' gaol and the blacking factory) may have conditioned his aloof attitude towards Overs. Together with his prejudices against Regency figures which will be discussed later, it may also lie behind his dismissive remarks on Clare. These were occasioned by reading Frederick Martin's *The Life of John Clare* which was published in 1865, one year after the poet's death. Martin certainly provides a lot of details for those who wanted to attack aristocratic and gentry forms of patronage, even if some individual patrons such as Radstock are exempted from his critique. He suggests that the local grandees could and should have done more for Clare. Marianne Marsh is (mis)represented as a batty eccentric who expects poets to be even more so. By this time, however, Clare was perhaps inextricably although unfairly connected with old-style patronage. The biography also provides new material that could be used against him. His prose writings, which might have interested social critics obsessed by fact, are written off as being poor, perhaps because Martin wants to assert his own shaky credentials as a prose writer. Clare's descriptive abilities (Holywell Hall, Byron's funeral, the Londoners, his patrons and many other examples not used here) are being badly underrated, as is his ability in his letters to find memorable words and phrases. To be fair to Martin, he reproduces Clare's account of his escape from the first asylum and quotes from letters, mainly to Taylor and Cunningham. He nevertheless quotes surprisingly little of the earlier poetry. Perhaps most damaging of all, Clare's drinking is presented as having been a problem at various points during his literary life, which self-consciously went against the grain of Victorian literary biographies that sought to be keepers of a sacred flame and were thus often economical with the truth about the allegedly private vices of public figures. Martin may indeed go to the other extreme and exaggerate Clare's dependency on drink, or at least not set out an appropriate context for it.

Clare and John, sometimes more deferentially Sir John, Barleycorn certainly had a very troubled love–hate relationship. Perhaps Clare was right to predict that Barleycorn, whose name may be taken from Burns's 'Tam O' Shanter' as well as from folk sources, 'will turn a skulking masterly foe at the end' (*LJC*, p. 79). He went on some very big benders indeed, for instance on his way back from London in 1822, and when he went to Boston in 1828. As noted, his publishers and patrons voiced the kind of evangelical objections to his drinking that were to underpin Victorian temperance movements and, as will be seen later, contributed to the idea of moral insanity. Martin's account runs the risk of making him appear to be a throwback to the bad old days of Regency permissiveness. The high society excesses of this period are well known: a valet (Carlyle's nightmare) advised his aristocratic master, at a loss to know what to wear to yet another boring masquerade ball, to surprise absolutely everybody including himself and go sober. Clare himself documents throughout his autobiographical writings the way in which drink lubricated the work and leisure of labourers during the Regency. The life of the gardeners at Burghley revolved around drink and the Stamford fair provided an annual occasion to get very fresh indeed, to use one of his own expressions. Evangelical voices like those of Radstock and the Vice Society may have been increasingly raised against such practices and yet they were also still widely tolerated. For large parts of Regency society, nothing succeeded like excess. Many soldiers and sailors went into battle either roaring drunk, or else extremely hungover. Many successful prize-fighters, who were Clare's heroes, often hit the brandy before, during and after a bout. A boxer called Dutch Sam, who will be considered very briefly later, always turned up drunk. Talking of brandy, Clare toasted one of his correspondents with brandy and water during the Christmas of 1828 (*LJC*, p. 449) and then told Taylor a few days later that he had not touched spirits for years (*LJC*, p. 451). There is certainly some denial in his letters, although his drinking still needs to be related to both his period and his class.

The evidence is not always easy to recover, but it still seems likely that Clare's associations with Regency excess, emphasised but not sufficiently explained by Martin, may not have particularly endeared him to eminently Victorian readers. The *London Magazine* group or coterie could resist anything but temptation. Lamb had actually been placed in the stocks for drinking on a Sunday. He had timed his saturnalia amiss! Sabbitarianism, it will be remembered, was one of the agendas of SSV. Although De Quincey claimed to be an opium-eater he, like

Coleridge, usually preferred to drink a diluted version of his poison known as laudanum. Both of them were to claim that it was the drink rather than the drugs that was undermining them.[22] Perhaps this was also a form of denial. Many Victorian writers were not saints, but they often found biographers who allowed readers to believe that they might have been (Carlyle's biography was an exception to this rule). This may seem a harsh judgement on Martin, whose reasonably detailed research rescued Clare if not quite from oblivion then at least from obscurity.[23] A biography that struck the right notes at the right time could create almost single-handedly a literary reputation, as happened with Richard Monckton Milnes's study of Keats in 1848. Martin's biography did not have anything like this kind of impact.

Perhaps the literary prejudices against Clare, the day before yesterday's man, were just too deeply engrained for this ever to have been possible in the first place. Although Martin's study was followed in 1873 by J.L. Cherry's *Life and Remains of John Clare, The Northamptonshire Peasant Poet*, Clare's reputation remained a fringe one throughout the Victorian period. Cherry was much more complimentary than Martin had been about Clare's patrons and published in revised form some of the asylum poetry. It is possible that if Taylor, with his greater knowledge of Clare, had completed the collected works which he was contemplating in the 1850s, the poet's reputation might have been more secure. De Quincey's reputation certainly benefited from the publication of his collected works first in America and then in Britain. There was another edition of Clare's work, by Arthur Symons in 1908, but he did not figure at all prominently in the turn-of-the-century Regency revival (for instance, Wilde's interest in Wainewright, or the way in which Byron's reputation revived) because his connections with the *London Magazine* were not well documented. The pattern of his literary life after death had been more or less set. He and his reputation were not there to be explored in increasing detail but, more simply, to be discovered anew and afresh by editors, biographers, other writers and readers, and then celebrated. His neglect tended to be something that was not reconstructed historically by looking specifically at the transition from Regency to Victorian, but rather as a sad event to be treated more subjectively and emotionally. Drury, Gilchrist and Taylor told discovery narratives about Clare. So, until relatively recently, did some critics and editors.

All *you* would wish a poor man to be

A Scottish handloom weaver called William Thom was dramatically rescued from poverty in 1841 by James Gordon, a local landowner or laird with extensive business interests. Thom had published a poem, prefaced with an account of his hardship, in the local press. Gordon sent him sums of money and made enquiries about his circumstances. He was both relieved and bewildered by this sudden transition from extreme shade to bright sunshine, or what Clare called wearing into sunshine. He had, like Clare, no pastoral illusions about the supposed benefits of poverty and so was initially anxious to impress his new patron. He was quite happy to try to play the part of the deserving poor that was being scripted for him. He signed one of his letters 'All you would wish a poor man to be'.[24] He did not want to be 'lip-deep in poverty again'.[25]

Gordon advised against premature publication and explored the possibility that Thom might be trained to become a school teacher (as indicated there was some discussion of such training for Clare, until his bad habits put a stop to it). Gordon brought his poet to London in 1841, almost immediately after the dramatic discovery and intervention, to introduce him to the great and the good. The visit may be compared with Burns's first visit to Edinburgh and Clare's earlier trips to London. Gordon clearly believed in the virtues of dilettante patronage. He tried to persuade Thom to dedicate his poems to one of the fashionable ladies at court. It seems likely that he eventually presented a copy of them to Queen Victoria herself, who subscribed to the hardship fund for the poet's family in 1848. He also took the trouble to get his pet artisan invited to the salons of some of the most influential hostesses of the time such as Lady Blessington's at Gore House, where dandyism and valetism still reigned gloriously supreme despite the dominant cult of earnestness. She was the author of *Conversations with Lord Byron* (1834), as well as of silver-fork novels celebrating Regency high society. *Rhymes and Recollections of a Handloom Weaver*, expensively priced, was not published until 1844. The main reason for the delay, in addition to Thom's indolence and diffidence, was that Gordon took a long time to write the patron's text, which consisted of his own antiquarian notes together with translations of dialect words.

Thom sometimes represented himself to his friends as a victim of dilettante patronage, who was forced to dance a 'jig to the humours of a foolish patron'.[26] He claimed that Gordon had invited him to 'his mansion and made an heir of me, and then cast me off. I had too much independence for him, and he wanted me to grovel'.[27] Kingsley buys into this version of events when Mackaye tells Alton that the rich left Thom to die in a ditch. Although poet and patron certainly had the usual disagreements over access to money as experienced by Yearsley, Clare and many others, it is still unfair to lay all Thom's troubles at

Gordon's mansion door. Indeed Thom himself, like Clare, had an ambivalent attitude towards patronage. He may have sometimes sounded off against it in relatively private letters or conversations, whereas in more public statements he could acknowledge some of its undoubted benefits.

Although dilettante patronage delayed the publication of *Rhymes and Recollections* until the summer of 1844, its timing still turned out to be perfect. For the Burns Festival that took place then got a lot of people thinking about relationships between poetry and poverty, literature and labour. Some English journalists, notably Jerrold, seized on Thom's literary life as a way of highlighting the smug and safe nostalgia that both promoted and protected the Burns myth. Jerrold's first article in *Punch* urges Scotland to honour living poets like Thom as well as dead ones like Burns. A second article deals with Thom's life in some detail. Jerrold belonged to the radical Bohemia of the metropolis (which included the *Punch* group and Henry Mayhew) and had a reputation for wit and repartee. Yet his jokes often had a serious side too: 'earnest in the very wit with which he vented his sense of detestation for evil doing'.[28]

The literary pages of the main Chartist newspaper, *The Northern Star*, under the editorship of Julian Harney, also attacked the hypocrisy of the Burns cult: nostalgia for a dead poet and his shrine (which had been visited earlier by both Wordsworth and Keats), coupled with indifference to living ones. In addition to Thom's case for patronage, the claims of one of Burns's alleged daughters and Sarah Parker, a 'poor Irish girl' who wrote poetry, were also canvassed.[29] The cult of the butch artisan poet disadvantaged Clare himself, although not so severely as it did women writers from the same class who found publication harder in this period than in previous ones. There is no British equivalent of *The Lowell Offering*, the literary journal published by women factory workers in America in the early 1840s.[30]

Memories of Clare were revived by *The Northern Star* as part of this concerted campaign to expose the underside of the Burns cult. An article from *Berrow's Worcester Journal* was reprinted on 5 October 1844. It tells the story of a visit to the asylum to see Clare. The author (a journalist called John Noake) inspects the asylum and likes what he sees. He is told that he will find Clare underneath the colonnade of a local church. The poet is described as being 'habited in a fustian dress, and there was nothing in his appearance which would distinguish him from the ordinary race of peasants, except that on closer inspection his countenance still exhibited traces of that intellectual spirit which erewhile had lurked within'. Clare, seen as a peasant rather than as a labourer, is addicted both to his pipe and to 'delusions' that he is 'the best pugilist in the kingdom'. His poetry is seen as being of variable quality: 'His style is now very uncertain, and always tinctured by that of the last author he has read. Sometimes his poetry is unworthy of the name, being coarse and vulgar; at others it is very beautiful.' Despite the increasing emphasis on the sturdy virtues of earnest artisan poets, it is just possible that there could have been a significant revival of interest in Clare in 1844 as a result of these heated debates about the patronage of humble poets. Yet this article, while certainly giving him some publicity, also shows why this was not the case. His confinement in the asylum meant that he tended to be presented as a pathetic figure, even though this image can in fact be constructed only by dismissing the alleged coarseness, and therefore vitality, of some of his writings, together with his pugnacious behaviour. It will be argued later that the pugilistic performances, far from being a sign of madness, might have been a perfectly coherent way for him to carry on reading the riddles of his Regency literary life. The quest, however, was on for living poets and his apparent madness placed him somewhere between the living and the dead. His death was in fact announced by *The Times* on 17 June 1840.

To return briefly to Thom, Jerrold was at one level clearly using him cynically to attack the Burns myth and yet he also took trouble to befriend the poet. He wrote to John Forster, the editor of *The Examiner*, later in 1844 to advise him what to do with the money that was being sent in there for Thom's benefit: 'His views are very humble, and judging from what he has written to me, he seems really to have written his true self in his book.'[31] A review of the book in *The Examiner* agrees with this view: 'The rhymes are to be read with interest and not without admiration: there being an earnest truth in them which shapes itself into words of beauty; a cry of real suffering which has broken into song.' The review reiterates the almost standard early Victorian critique of earlier, Regency forms of patronage: 'It was the fashion some years ago to patronise the poetry of housekeepers, butlers, and dairymaids; and a very unwholesome fashion it was...It is however no wail of neglected genius raised in this book of Mr Thom's, but a cry that more nearly concerns us all. Is the deeply seated disease from which it comes to be left for ever without a remedy?' (14 September 1844, pp. 380–1). Thom was presented as speaking for his class rather than making a special case for his own personal advancement.

Almost all the reviews hail Thom as an earnest, sincere speaker of the truth. *The Reasoner* claims that he had 'produced a *genuine* book – a book, which, as it is the record of a *real life*, and written in a *sincere* and impassioned style, so it is a solemn warning to society, that it is built on dangerous ground, pregnant with the perils of injustice' (2, p. 39). *The Illuminated Magazine* praises him for speaking the whole truth and nothing but the truth: 'We have no fiction here; no fabrication of artificial woes; every emotion recorded has been felt; every pang has been suffered.' This review goes on to strike an even more Carlylean tone when it declares that the poet must provide the kind of vital, essential information that was missing from government reports. It is worth quoting at some length since it articulates many of the assumptions in this period which prevented Clare from being given a fair hearing:

> It is a revelation of the 'woes unnumbered' under which thousands – nay, millions – of our fellow-beings are doomed to struggle through existence. The individual instance is but a type of many; but the many have not the power of giving their sorrows voice; they suffer in silence, and pass away unheard; and but for the few – the very few, who, like William Thom, can throw the feelings and thoughts of his class into a form and language that can win their way to the hearts of all – those who move in what are called the upper circles of society, would be almost entirely ignorant of the condition of the labouring portion of their fellow-countrymen, as if they were divided from them by oceans or spoke another tongue. They would only know of their existence by the figures of statistical tables, or the 'Reports' of Poor-Law Commissioners, which, dealing only with the masses, and giving only numerical results, become mere mathematical abstractions, and keep out of sight everything like individual or human emotion. Of this, such a book as the present, is a corrective. (4, p. 50)

Thom's primary function is to provide earnest sages with qualitative, emblematic and essential information about the state of the nation, and to do it fast.

The social critics who patronised Thom burdened him with great expectations that were destined to remain unrealised. Jerrold continued to cite the poet's experiences as a way of authenticating his own reforming agenda. An article in *The Shilling Magazine* on 'The Temptations of the Poor' invokes Thom's authority: 'Let it not be thought that this picture is over-drawn for the purpose of palliating the crimes of the poor. It is coloured by the hand of truth ... The simple but forcible narrative of the weaver Thom ... will illustrate its truth' (1, pp. 444–5).

The problem was that, after the delayed publication of *Rhymes and Recollections*, Thom did not produce anything else that made the desired significant, sustained contribution to social debates. One of the reasons for this was that his patrons, like Clare's, did not want him to become a professional writer. Thus, for a time, he was encouraged to establish himself as a linen-weaver in London, using his popularity to solicit orders. Just as Clare/Percy Green had been encouraged at times to dress up very self-consciously in an old-fashioned peasant's costume, so Thom played the theatrical role that was scripted for him. He became a token artisan, paradoxically trying to pursue the trade of customary weaving which his own writings had shown to be in terminal decline. Another reason why he failed to live up to the great expectations was that his patrons wanted him to be a journalist or at least a prose writer, while he was much more concerned with writing songs and reworking traditional texts. He may have been heavily promoted as a new kind of artisan-writer, yet his roots always lay in an older vernacular tradition. Clare, who was Scottish on his father's side, felt that 'scotch Poets' (*BH*, p. 185) were often at their best when producing and reproducing songs rather than poems, which could be self-conscious and affected.

It has been possible to notice some similarities between Thom's patronage in the 1840s and Clare's reception in the 1820s. Yet there were also some fundamental differences between Regency and early Victorian attitudes towards working-class writers. Thom may have actually been discovered by a dilettante patron, but as suggested his popularity depended on the way in which his life and work could be incorporated into topical debates over the Condition-of-England question. It was not just middle-class radicals like Jerrold who attempted to recruit him to their own particular crusades. A number of Chartists, notably Harney, befriended him in the hope that he would champion their particular cause and it is clear that he had some sympathies with more advanced forms of radicalism. It may be that he was a little bit too anxious to try to please all of his real and potential patrons, to be all that everybody would wish a poor man to be. The problem with this was that each group ultimately had different and competing agendas. Clare was much better at remaining friends with those on opposing political sides.

Thom died in Dundee in 1848 not, as Kingsley would have it, the victim of old-fashioned patronage with its glass birdcages but rather because he often found himself trapped in contradictory positions as a result of trying to please all of his patrons all of the time. The cult of the artisan-poet as promoted by Carlyle and his followers emphasised vigour and strength, and often contained a submerged homo-erotic script. Ironically, many of the poets who were discovered (often like Clare when they were relatively old) were almost complete physical wrecks as a result of trying to combine literature and labour. For Thom and some others the ravages of early poverty and injury were made worse by a fondness for that crafty old devil Barleycorn. For a variety of reasons one has to look elsewhere for literary celebrations of artisan values, perhaps to Walt Whitman's *Leaves of Grass* (1855) and to some of George Eliot's novels such *Adam Bede* (1859) and *Felix Holt the Radical* (1866).

A backbone of personal experience

Samuel Bamford had also been a handloom weaver. He marketed himself as a 'weaver boy' poet when both Keats and Clare were trying to establish themselves. It has been suggested that Clare, who always took a keen interest as has been seen in poets from his own class, might have read and been influenced by extracts from Bamford in a Stamford newspaper at this time (EP, 1, pp. xv–vi). Bamford's later autobiographical publications, *Passages in the Life of a Radical* (1839/41) and *Early Days* (1848/9) brought him to the notice of those who struggled to give utterance to answers the Condition-of-England question. He had been imprisoned after Peterloo (the conversion narrative again), and his politics became more gradualist and therefore acceptable to middle-class patrons. He claims that his writings filled an important gap: 'the real condition of the people was not understood, by those above them, who only sought a knowledge of them from information derived from magistrates, parsons, ladies, ladies maids, poor law officers & such like.'[32] This claim, and the misogyny that went with it, was accepted without too many qualifications by the sages. Carlyle urged Bamford to carry on contributing essential information 'about Lancashire operatives, and their ways of living and thinking, their miseries and advantages, their virtues and sins'. He threw in a reminder that 'Fact is eternal; all fiction is very transitory in comparison'.[33] He warned him that the spirit of this earnest age did not favour the publication of poetry. *The Examiner* admired Bamford's earnestness and sincerity more than it did his poetry. *The Athenaeum* praised his writing for correcting at a stroke the 'misjudging representations' about the working class that were in circulation: 'it reveals to us more of the mind of the operatives in the manufacturing districts, their intellectual condition, their moral principles, and their social feelings, than we are likely to obtain from any other source.'[34]

Just as Kingsley used Cooper to add authenticity to *Alton Locke*, so other writers appropriated Bamford's life and work to add an aura of truth to their own fictions. William Howitt's *The Man of the People* (1860), which deals with radicalism between 1815 and 1819, draws heavily on Bamford's writings and Bamford himself is introduced as a character, albeit a minor one. Clare was visited in the asylum by Mary Howitt in 1844 and then by William in 1846. Sir James Kay-Shuttleworth was a leading social reformer, particularly associated with education. He wrote to Bamford in 1859: 'I have several times read your life of a Radical, & have just read a second time your "Early Days", I have much to say to you.'[35] Bamford immediately retrieved his coat from the pawnbroker's shop and hastily beat a path to the door of Kay-Shuttleworth's mansion: 'very cordially received by Sir James, who told me he wanted the information he had written about, in order to show (in a publication, as I understood) the influence of education on the conduct of working men, as exhibited in their strikes, riots & other popular demonstrations'.[36] Bamford started to research the subject and Kay-Shuttleworth seemed very pleased with the results, claiming that he was the ideal source of information because '*From you*, such a work, would have a "*backbone*" of personal experience, or observation'.[37] Manly artisans not only had backbone themselves, but also provided it for others.

Kay-Shuttleworth paid Bamford for his work and also tried to promote his interests more generally. Bamford was never quite sure how and where his information was going to be used. It ultimately formed the '*backbone*' to Kay-Shuttleworth's social-problem novel *Scarsdale* (1860). Bamford spotted his own contributions when he read the novel. Besides the actual descriptions of strikes, he noted that many of the topographical details were similar to passages in his own work.

The Reverend William Gaskell's obituary in *The Manchester Guardian* on 12 June 1884 noted that '*The Poets of Humble Life*; *The Poetry of Thomas Hood*; *Samuel Bamford* and *The Lancashire Dialect* were a few of his favourite subjects'. These were all topics on which he had lectured either at the Working Men's College, or else at Mechanics' Institutes. He was particularly interested in Bamford's attempts to preserve Lancashire dialect. Bamford's work in this area is mentioned at the beginning of *Two Lectures on the Lancashire Dialect*, which formed an appendix to the fifth edition of Elizabeth Gaskell's *Mary Barton* in 1854. Although Bamford's work is certainly acknowledged here, it is possible that his

Dialect of South Lancashire (1850) provided more of a '*backbone*' to these lectures than was indicated. Both men shared an admiration for 'Tim Bobbin' (or John Collier), the eighteenth-century Lancashire dialect writer. Bamford saw himself as Bobbin's unacknowledged successor, and bitterly lamented the fact that he had never been given the opportunities and resources to conduct a thorough study of Lancashire dialect. When he was shown a copy of William Gaskell's two lectures he detected some inaccuracies in them, even though he was in general terms impressed by them. Similarly, in an otherwise effusive and supportive letter to Elizabeth Gaskell following the first publication of *Mary Barton* in 1848, he pointed out that the dialect could have been improved.

Bamford was something of a local celebrity. Carlyle and Jane Welsh Carlyle were taken to meet him when they visited Manchester, as were other social tourists. Residents like the Gaskells were in contact with him at this time as well. Elizabeth wrote to Forster to see if he could persuade Tennyson to provide Bamford with copies of his poetry. She gave Forster a quick thumbnail sketch: 'A great, gaunt, stalwart Lancashire man, formerly hand-loom weaver, author of "Life of a Radical" &c – age nearly 70, and living in that state which is exactly "decent poverty".'[38] Ten years later Bamford complained to his dear diary that he had, at some point, been unceremoniously dumped as an acquaintance by William Gaskell.[39] The diary is full of charges of neglect, some no doubt real but others imaginary. The tone, more generally, is peevish and tetchy. Bamford, trying to eke out a precarious living as a performance-poet, is cross that Dickens can attract large audiences in Manchester and is worried in case Cooper might also upstage him. Public performances offered some sort of a lifeline to working-class writers, mostly unable to join the literary profession and yet reluctant to resume their previous occupations. This made sense, however, only in Manchester and other large cities like Sheffield, which could deliver audiences. Although Clare played the fiddle at local gatherings, he may well have been too shy to have gone into performance in a big way. Yet situated as he was, this was never really a realistic option anyway. Peterborough did not get a Mechanics' Institute, a possible venue for him, until 1832. He turned down the invitation to give a speech at Boston in 1828. He had gone there, amongst other reasons, to try to sell copies of *The Shepherd's Calendar*. Other potential invitations, for instance to Hull, were not accepted. He could perhaps have eked out some sort of wandering literary life in East Anglia and adjacent areas, but only just. He was too shy to do this, but perhaps also too proud: he could and should have been as successful as Lord Byron. It was not a good combination. A letter to Taylor indicates that Clare spent some time in Boston talking about his acquaintance with Lamb and De Quincey (*LJC*, p. 441). He was dining out in Boston as a literary man with London connections rather than as the local folk singer. The same letter shows that he was reading and appreciating Virgil. Another letter, also to Taylor, indicates that the table-talk at Boston was about 'the Poets' (*LJC*, p. 450).

Bamford is referred to in *Mary Barton* itself as 'a man who illustrates his order and shows what nobility may be in a cottage'.[40] One of his poems, 'God Help the Poor', which recommends patience and fortitude in the face of adversity, is not just quoted in the novel but also performs a complicated plot function within it. His message of resignation counterpoints Chartist and trades union calls for retaliation. Although Gaskell does not use his life and works nearly as crudely as Kay-Shuttleworth was to do, it is still the case that they provided some of the '*backbone*' to her representations of Lancashire lives and languages, and her particular version of urban pastoral which recommends the re-establishment of cottage virtues and 'decent poverty' in this bleak new environment. This urban pastoral is articulated by a character called Alice Wilson who remains true to her rural roots. As so often in accounts of rural values in this period, the influences here are Wordsworth and George Crabbe rather than Clare. Wordsworthian Romanticism, which claims to speak on behalf of the rural labourers, has always tended from very early on to marginalise Clare. Gaskell's account of working-class values is, at times, refreshingly different from that championed by Carlyle. Whereas he sings the praises of rough and rugged masculinity she notices, particularly in the earlier parts of the novel, qualities of caring and sharing in John Barton that are eventually undermined by narcotics such as Chartism and opium that are seen as coming from outside the potentially pastoral community.[41]

Missed opportunities

The aim in this chapter has not been to provide anything like a comprehensive study of the reception of working-class writings in the early Victorian period. It has, rather, been to quote enough from reviews and other sources to establish the emergence of the new assumptions and vocabularies that worked to Clare's disadvantage. Even without the periods of illness followed by the long confinements in asylums, he would have found it increasingly difficult to please a public that had such clear and rigid expectations about the function, or utility, of working-class writers, as well as about the new type of patronage that was necessary.

As has been seen, Clare was not completely neglected since his experiences even if misunderstood could still be used in general terms to suggest improvements to the Condition-of-England. Edwin Paxton Hood, a supporter of self-help who took some trouble to research Clare's story, offered appreciations of him in *The Literature of Labour* (1851) and elsewhere. Hood nevertheless assumed that the story would not be widely known by his readers, even those who moved in literary circles. Some working-class poets continued to be inspired by Clare's example. Joseph Dare, one of a group of poets associated with Leicester, published a poem in his *The Garland of Gratitude* (1848), written after learning that Clare was confined in an asylum. One of the Manchester poets, Edwin Waugh, put a poem by Clare in his commonplace book. It has to be said, however, that Clare never started to compete with Burns as a source of inspiration for such writers. This is regrettable given the way in which he himself openly acknowledged, as has been seen, the influences of Burns, Bloomfield, Chatterton and Kirke White. More generally, Clare lived in Burns's shadow throughout the early Victorian period and beyond.[42] He admired Burns's poetry (if not his letters), although had much less time for 'the idolators of the Scottish bard' (*LJC*, p. 236). Many influential writers (such as Carlyle), journalists and publishers came from Scottish backgrounds. A Scottish mafia continued to dominate parts of the English literary scene and was concerned to promote the merits of their own countrymen. Burns was one of Carlyle's heroes in the lectures delivered in 1841 which became *On Heroes, Hero-Worship and the Heroic in History*. This is not to underestimate Burns's achievements, nor indeed to argue that Clare's merits have to be asserted at the expense of those of other writers. It is, rather, to notice some of the specifically historical reasons for Burns's prominence. An interest in his literary life might have led naturally to a concern to promote Clare as well, but for a variety of reasons, some of them connected with literary nationalism, this did not happen. Working-class writers continued to look to Burns rather than to Clare for inspiration. D.H. Lawrence, for example, made a start on a novel about Burns.[43] Literary nationalism also benefited Hogg, who was guest-of-honour at a Burns dinner in London in 1832. His writings on the supernatural, together with those of other writers from *Blackwood's*, influenced the Brontës as well as Gaskell (who was first published in *Blackwood's*). He had a much higher profile than Clare in Britain, as well as in America, as a result of Edgar Allan Poe's love–hate relationship with the *Blackwood's* style.[44] Clare, in keeping with the respect that he had always felt for poets from similar backgrounds, wanted to come to London in 1832 to meet Hogg (*LJC*, p. 574). He claimed to like everything that the Etterick Shepherd had written (*LJC*, p. 633). Through his correspondence with George Reid, he was able to develop his interest in Scottish writers.

Clare's name is sometimes included in the litanies of humble geniuses by Smiles (for example, in a biography of a French barber-poet) and others that formed an important part of self-help literature, although it is more often than not conspicuous by its absence.[45] Like some of Clare's own poetry, it is the range of the catalogue which is important here. It would have defeated the object of exemplary biographies to have singled out any one individual genius for special attention. It is the sheer number of examples that makes the most telling point. Clare may sometimes get a mention, but then it is time to move quickly on to the next example.

Cyrus Redding, himself a Regency relic, published long accounts of Clare in the *English Journal* after visiting him in the asylum. Yet Clare's agricultural background and passion for pastoral poetry did not endear him to many of those who wrote on social issues which were seen as being primarily urban, and indeed sometimes specifically metropolitan. His associations with aristocratic patrons did not help his cause, nor did his links with some Regency values and lifestyles that were increasingly being seen as old-fashioned. There was, however, much wishful thinking surrounding the emerging cult of the artisan-poet in the early Victorian period. Like Clare, both Thom and Bamford were preoccupied with old rural customs, as well as with the uses of dialect. Some of Elliott's best poetry is in the pastoral tradition. The idea, or ideal, of the artisan-poet was often very different from the reality. Some of them, far from following the script by becoming earnest and original tellers of the truth, were more interested in demonstrating their familiarity with existing poetic conventions. Others remained rooted in folk traditions.

Clare's popularity was not helped, however, by the fact that some of his writings which might have interested the new breed of patrons remained unpublished in book-form. Social criticism such as 'The Parish', as well as many of his attempts to reproduce folk songs, were unavailable in book-form. Although it seems unlikely that Dickens would ever have been convinced of Clare's merits despite the fact that there are some similarities between their language-games, there were others such as Kingsley who were passionately interested, in theory anyway, in the songs of the people and might have been persuaded of Clare's continuing importance had the evidence been available. Clare had begun collecting 'National and Provincial Melodies' in the 1820s with a view to publication. It was an impressive collection, ahead of its time.[46] Thom's *Recollections* and Bamford's *Passages* and *Early Days* were by no means the only working-class autobiographies that attracted attention in this period: Alexander Somerville (ploughboy), Christopher Thomson (artisan) and W.D. Burn (beggarboy) also gained notice.[47] Yet Clare's autobiographical writings remained unpublished. His 'Journal' which, as indicated earlier, shows the depth of his reading, was also not available. *Mary Barton* includes an affectionate study of a working-class naturalist, patient old Job Legh. Clare's prose writings on the natural history of Helpston were not available. This is not to say that Clare's claim to attention should have rested primarily on his prose rather than his poetry, but to suggest that its publication might have resulted in more interest in him during a period that was obsessed by the languages of fact. He wrote sympathetically and knowledgably about gypsy life. He may have seriously considered joining this world at one point, and gypsies gave him the idea of escaping from the High Beach asylum. There are representations of gypsies in 'The Village Minstrel', *The Shepherd's Calendar* and elsewhere. Yet Clare does not seem to have benefited from the popularity of George Borrow's work on gypsies.[48] As so often, the opportunities for a revival of interest were missed. There were many potential turning points about which his reputation did not in the event turn.

As noticed earlier, some of Clare's dialect words and expressions were edited out by John Taylor's pruning hook. The cultural climate in the 1840s was much more receptive towards such writing: William Barnes's dialect poetry was first published in 1844. Although a dominant image is of Clare as a nostalgic writer this should not, given the riddles of pastoral, rule out the possibility that he was also capable at one and the same time of anticipating cultural developments. Pastoral yearns for the past, and yet also comments on the present and provides programmes for the future. Clare had collaborated on *A Glossary of Northamptonshire Words and Places* which was eventually published in 1853 and included some examples from unpublished asylum poetry as well as many others from his published work. Put at its very simplest, the Condition-of-England question asked what might unite those who appeared to be dangerously divided economically from each other. One very widely canvassed answer was to suggest that there was a common language and therefore culture. Gaskell's footnotes in *Mary Barton* are designed to show that, despite the seeming inaccessibility of Lancashire dialect to outsiders, it nevertheless often had its origins in Anglo-Saxon usage as well as in Chaucerian English. Tradition provided respectability. Clare anticipated some of these arguments, noticing that Chaucerian vocabulary was still 'very common now in what is called the mouths of the vulgar though sometimes used differently as to meaning' (*LJC*, p. 547). Tim Bobbin had also been influenced by Chaucerian English. The desire to build unity through a shared sense of Saxondom was a dominant theme in the works of Paxton Hood and others. Some writers, notably Carlyle, were much more explicitly racist in the ways in which they extolled what were seen to be the virtues of a national and international Teutonic brotherhood, and it was this racism that eventually contributed to the narrowing of the broadly based support and influence that he had enjoyed in the early Victorian period. Clare's writings might perhaps have made some contribution to such debates about the possibility of a common language, if they had not been tidied up during the 1820s and 1830s. As it was, however, they did not provide in their published form enough material to encourage further research and interest.

Some of the reasons for Clare's neglect must remain speculative. There can, however, be less room for doubt about the way in which his confinement in asylums from 1837 until his death in 1864 contributed to his neglect. It is therefore necessary to move on to reconstruct the world of the asylum and place Clare and his work within it. Although it will be seen that there were attempts by those who pioneered a method of treatment known as moral management to remove the stigma that was attached to madness they were, at best, only partially successful. The perception of Clare as being mad probably did more damage than anything else to his reception and reputation. It meant, and often still does mean, that the most favourable reaction that could be expected was sentimental pity for his pathetic condition. As will be seen, however, there are thankfully other responses that can be taken to the asylum period, one of which is to ask what he was doing there in the first place.

4
High, Flighty and Frolicsome: Mad Poets and Moral Managers

Life sentences

Clare spent over a quarter of a century confined in lunatic asylums. He was placed first of all in the High Beach Asylum in Epping Forest in June 1837, paid for by a subscription fund. Eliza Emmerson gave five pounds. Clare's occupation is listed as labourer first, and then poet: the story of his literary life once again in nutshell. This was a private asylum run by Matthew Allen according to new ideas on moral management, which will be explained during the course of the chapter. Clare escaped in 1841 and walked almost all the way back home. After a short break, he was then placed in the Northamptonshire General Lunatic Asylum, paid for by Earl Fitzwilliam. Although not strictly speaking a county asylum, this nevertheless had some affinities with such institutions. He served a 'life sentence' in asylums, and then some more.[1] His experiences, over this long period, will be related to other life stories of the allegedly insane sometimes told in their own words and sometimes told by the authorities. As mentioned right at the beginning of this book, no claim is being made that Clare either knew or was influenced by such stories. The argument is once again that Clare's own story can be illuminated by other ones.

This chapter explores the origins and growth of asylum culture in the Regency and early Victorian periods, concentrating to some extent on the Quaker York Retreat which was seen as pioneering moral management techniques. A number of those who had charge of Clare were inspired by its example. High Beach was modelled on it and Thomas Prichard, the first Medical Superintendent at Northampton, tried to introduce aspects of moral management there even though it did not transfer well to larger institutions with a high percentage of working-class inmates. As suggested, Clare's publishers and patrons were involved in a form of moral management in the 1820s, particularly trying to get him to give up the demon drink. He was eventually handed over to those who claimed to be professionals in this field.

Moral management thrived best in an affluent environment. Its demise was hastened not just by the increasing medicalisation of asylum culture, but also by the rapid expansion in numbers from the early Victorian period onwards. Although a County Asylums Act had been passed in 1808, it was not followed by an extensive building programme. This happened only after the passing of the Lunatic Asylums Act in 1845. Unlike the Retreat, the new county asylums were increasingly flooded with those from the poorer sections of society. These inmates often reached the asylum only after being held for long periods of time in other institutions such as workhouses either as lunatics or just as paupers, and were seen as being incurable. It was, perhaps, their institutionalisation rather than their alleged madness that was beyond cure. Clare claims that his early attempts to acquire an education through reading encouraged the villagers to see him as destined to become 'an idiot for a workhouse' (*AW*, p. 5), a point that is also made as has been seen in 'The Fate of Genius'. As far as perceptions of him were and are concerned, in a way these villagers may have been right. The pioneers of moral management had advocated small numbers, together with a policy of early admission. Their methods also depended on an ability to employ a large number of trained attendants. None of these essential conditions was to be found in the county asylums, or in institutions such as the Northamptonshire General Lunatic Asylum, which in the Victorian period developed essentially custodial rather than curative functions. Those with money, such as Mr Dick in Dickens's *David Copperfield* (1849–50), could keep themselves out of asylums. Those with supportive and tolerant friends, such as Miss Bates in Austen's *Emma*, were cared for within the community. The poor often found it harder to avoid the clutches of the mad-doctors.

Two specific themes will be highlighted here, in addition to the general aim of recovering and reconstructing asylum culture. First of all, it will be shown why the writing of poetry, and the uses of imagination more generally, were actively discouraged in the new asylums. This may help to explain why Clare wrote relatively little (that has survived) during the earlier part of his confinement at High Beach. As will be seen, prejudices against poetry were gradually replaced by more tolerant attitudes. As happened throughout his literary life, Clare was caught between different worlds. Second, it will be argued that Michel Foucault's influential view in *Madness and Civilisation* (1965) that there was no longer any dialogue between reason and unreason in the asylums is mistaken. As a prelude to analysing some of Clare's own asylum writings and pugilistic performances in the next chapter, it will be suggested that there were indeed opportunities for inmates to stage performances as a way of contesting their confinement. Asylum culture is shown to be highly theatrical. Dialogue can be performed, as well as spoken and written.

Scraps of poetry

Samuel W. was an inmate at the York Retreat from 1803 until his death in 1824. He was one of the richer inmates, having his own sitting-room and servant (what sort of life can that have been?). Many of the inmates at High Beach brought their servants with them, which must have made Clare even more conscious of his own lowly social position. Samuel W. wanted to be taken seriously as a poet, but his keepers were extremely suspicious of his literary activities and ambitions. He had clearly mistaken his identity. He was visited by a cousin at the beginning of 1807 and the two of them explored the neighbourhood together. According to the case-notes compiled by George Jepson, the Superintendent at the Retreat, this visit began to upset the balance of Samuel W.'s mind: 'During the course of the day, he was talkative frequently whispering to people, showing scraps of poetry, a certain wildness in the eyes, and flushing of the face.'[2] After his cousin had departed, he had what was described as a 'paroxysm' which lasted, on and off, for nearly a month.

Samuel W. was brought to the Retreat, apparently with his own consent, from Alton in Hampshire. He had previously been confined for short periods in a private madhouse in London. He was described on admission as being 'a widower aged 43' who 'became first deranged about 12 years ago'. Although it was stated that his illness was connected with 'unrequited love', he was also seen as somebody who was suffering from an hereditary condition.[3] Given that Quakers were forbidden to 'marry out' until 1860, many other inmates were also seen as being mad for love. It was obviously not just Quakers who were deemed to be madly in love. A number of Hazlitt's friends such as Benjamin Haydon felt that he had actually driven himself completely and utterly mad over Sarah Walker, and many readers of *Liber Amoris* (1823) have reached the same conclusion.[4] Branwell Brontë finally flipped when rejected by his Mrs Robinson, and so on. In fiction jilted women such as Miss Havisham in Dickens's *Great Expectations* (1860–1) lose their reason. Jepson's diagnosis as a whole should still be treated cautiously, even though it is true that two of Samuel W.'s sisters were also confined at the Retreat. Medical men and others in this period often described cases that baffled them as being hereditary in origin. The medical men who certified Clare in 1841 believed that his condition was hereditary, although aggravated or excited by his addiction to poetry. Poetry and addiction are connected yet again.

Jepson was a self-educated apothecary, who had little or no experience of treating mental illnesses before coming to the Retreat. His methods of diagnosis, although often primitive and extremely dogmatic even by the standards of the time, still followed the conventions by making a distinction between 'predisposing' and 'exciting' causes.[5] In addition to forms of religious and political enthusiasm, Jepson categorised intemperance and sexual desire, which he sometimes described as 'lustiveness', as being among the most prominent 'exciting' causes.[6] Such categorisation implied an idea of what was to become known in the 1830s, as a result of work by James Cowles Prichard and others, as moral insanity. His claim was that there were forms of insanity which had no identifiable, 'predisposing' cause and which were therefore entirely the result of what was seen to be a degenerate, disorderly and dissolute lifestyle.[7] Baffling and bewildering Barleycorn could drive you mad alone and unaided. The Chaplain at the Northampton Asylum pronounced unequivocally in 1856 (despite the lack of any medical qualifications whatsoever) that 'insanity was occasioned by whatsoever promoted vice, or was opposed to virtue, as by drunkenness, dissipation, infidel and revolutionary principles'.[8] Perhaps Clare was actually forced to listen to him spouting this reactionary nonsense. The counter-revolutionary ideas that some of Clare's patrons such as Radstock had voiced in the 1820s were now acquiring putative scientific justifications. Asylums became committed to the suppression and repression of vice.

Whether or not Clare had to listen to such sermons, there were certainly times when he got very angry indeed about organised religion. Writing to his wife Patty in either 1849 or 1850, he explodes: 'truth is truth & the rights of man – age of reason & common sense are sentences full of meaning & the best comment of its truth is themselves – an honest man makes priestcraft an odious lyar & coward & filthy disgrace to Christianity – that coward I hate & detest – the Revelations has a placard in capitals about 'The Whore of Babylon & the mother of Harlots' does it mean Priestcraft I think that it must' (*LJC*, p. 669). At the beginning of this tirade he lists three of Tom Paine's best-known works (*Rights of Man, Age of Reason* and *Common Sense*), and more generally takes up a Paineite position against priestcraft. As mentioned earlier, Radstock had tried to stop Paineite ideas undermining his authority in Newfoundland. Publishers of Paine were successfully prosecuted by both the Proclamation Society and the Vice Society. In the asylum Clare no longer has to pretend to be the man that Radstock wanted him to be.

The sexes were usually strictly segregated in asylums which made certain forms of 'lustiveness' such as heterosexual sex difficult if not completely impossible. There were occasionally recorded instances in Regency asylums of male attendants taking what were described as liberties with female inmates. Dirty talk was often recorded in case-notes but, beyond this, the documentation starts becoming evasive and reticent. It will come as no surprise to those who already know some of Clare's asylum poetry that his own case-notes record the use of 'both profane & filthy language'.[9] According to Mr Rochester, nobody could compete with his first wife when it came to foul language.

Anne Matthewman, aged 36, was brought from London by her husband and placed in the Lincoln Asylum in 1835, a couple of months after the birth of a stillborn child. Perhaps she was just very sad rather than mad. She remained at Lincoln for just under eight months, despite making it abundantly clear from the outset that this was against her will. When she was not listened to, she started to plot her escape. She made a break for it one evening, only to be partially restrained by one of the nurses. She nevertheless floored this nurse with what the House-Surgeon describes as a blow of 'such force as to throw her over the flower bed'. Pugilism was one way of hitting back at the authorities. The House-Surgeon just happens to spy Matthewman the next day apparently planning another escape route: 'I have little doubt that it is the intention of this patient to escape if possible – today she has been examining the walls and doors of the convalescent airing court.' She makes another attempt about a month later, calmly trying to walk out through one of the main entrances. She very nearly succeeds. It is at this point that her conduct starts becoming lustive. The Surgeon orders solitary confinement after she has been 'so lascivious and indecent in her conduct'. Later references speak of her 'very obscene and indecent manner'. There are fears that her conduct may be contagious and excite others. She is clearly doing more than just talking smut, as it is her manner and conduct, or behaviour, that are causing such panic and alarm. The mad-doctors created figures known as erotomaniacs, melancholic women who apparently often developed sexual crushes on male authority-figures. Matthewman behaves in a much more assertive, aggressive manner. Unless she is restrained and isolated, lustive lunatics might take over the asylum.[10]

The documentation provides no further details. There are a number of possible explanations. Matthewman could have been having a sexual relationship with one of the other women inmates. Clare's asylum writings draw attention to same-sex relationships. High Beach is represented as a place 'Where lady sods & buggers dwell / To play the dirty game' (*LP*, 1, p. 37). Dirty, which may be Clare's term for forms of homosexuality, also occurs in some of his other asylum writings. For instance in 'Child Harold' the asylum is represented as a place that contains 'Things here too dirty for the light of day / For in a madhouse there exists no law – ' (*LP*, 1, p. 46). Clare also describes the asylum world as the 'Land of sodom' (*LJC,* p. 657). There are enough other references to same-sex relationships for them to be read literally, as well as more rhetorically within a biblical context. 'Dirty' is used as a general term of abuse in earlier poems such as 'The Parish', but may acquire more precise meanings in the asylum. Asylum inmates often had to be restrained from tearing up their clothes and cavorting around naked, exposing their persons as it was occasionally put. There are a few recorded cases of genital mutilation. Masturbation, along with same-sex relationships, dare not speak its name too explicitly in early asylum records, particularly as far as women were concerned. It becomes more openly discussed by medical men a bit later on when a brutal form of corrective surgery known as clitoridectomy (first performed in private clinics rather than in asylums) was introduced. Fears of masturbation driving the mad even madder nevertheless haunted the early asylum superintendents and house-surgeons. Rich inmates like Samuel W. may have had their own sitting-rooms, but were not allowed to sleep on their own. Anyone who wanted to spend time on their own was suspected of being up to no good.

Returning to Matthewman, despite the evasiveness in the records it is perhaps the case that she was just planning a different kind of escape route. If she behaved really badly, and perhaps more importantly encouraged others to do the same, then there was a chance that she might be sent away before too much damage could be done. Or it may just have been the case that being lustive, performing and parading one's sexuality, was one way of contesting the authority of chaplains, medical men and husbands. It was how you stayed sane inside their insanity. Matthewman's departure does not seem to have allowed Lincoln to clean up its act. The Lunacy Commissioners heard complaints from female inmates in 1846 about obscenity and indecency. A flasher, an inmate rather than an attendant, had apparently been exposing his person.

Jepson believed that Samuel W.'s condition was always in danger of being aggravated by too much contact with the outside world. This is why he became concerned when Samuel W. was very 'talkative' towards the end of his cousin's visit in 1807. The case-notes begin with the diagnosis that 'paroxysms coming on may be perceived by his becoming inquisitive, repeating verses, and imitating preaching, and a peculiar cast, and winking with one eye, and they are preceded by sleepless nights'.[11] Jepson was worried whenever Samuel W. went off on a shop-till-you-drop spree. Samuel W. appears to have enjoyed giving Jepson the slip. He got up very early one morning in 1809 and led the Superintendent a merry dance before he was eventually recaptured. It was a manic game of hide-and-seek.

Jepson's literal-minded record of these danger signals misses the way in which Samuel W.'s actions probably carried a theatrical parody of discipline at the Retreat. The alleged madman's 'inquisitive' looks might well have been mimicking the Superintendent's own beady-eyed methods of surveillance. The case-notes for 1806 record that Samuel W. had been 'very busy about other people's affairs, finding fault with the conduct of one, vilifying another, prying and watching'.[12] Jepson himself had to pry and watch in order to compile such entries and perhaps offers an exaggerated representation of his own methods when he describes Samuel W.'s antic disposition.

Roy Porter suggests a broadly similar interpretation when he considers the relationship between John Haslam, the apothecary at Bedlam, and an inmate there called James Tilly Matthews. Haslam published *Illustrations of Madness* (1810) to show that there was no case at all for listening to pleas for Matthews to be released: he needed to be locked up and the key thrown away. Haslam felt that all he had to do was to provide readers with examples of Matthews' intricate and elaborate conspiracy theories to illustrate incurable madness. Matthews certainly had a particularly vivid imagination. He had been imprisoned in France during the earlier stages of the Revolution there and was very lucky to have escaped with his life. He believed on his release that he alone was qualified to mediate between the British and French governments. His will to power was not to become Napoleon but, rather, to have such leaders actually come to him for advice. It is not surprising that after his experiences in revolutionary France he continued to feel the presence of spies 'before me, behind me and on every side of me' throughout his life.[13] This was a specifically political form of paranoia, which Porter suggests was shared by many establishment figures in the 1790s such as Edmund Burke who, to unriddle it just a bit, was paradoxically himself in many respects the enemy that he warned so vehemently against. Home Office papers reveal that this form of paranoia was also common amongst British radicals given the government's espionage system: identities on both sides were often merely theatrical disguises.[14] William Godwin's *Caleb Williams* (1794) explores both these related forms of political paranoia. Matthews drew heavily, and eclectically, on various new scientific developments. He imagines his omnipresent but often invisible enemies building elaborate and intricate machines to ensnare him, as well as being in the business of thought-transference. Porter suggests that he might have been representing the activities of Haslam himself in his descriptions of mechanical, as well as mental, torture: 'Haslam described Matthews in print. But in doing so, he perhaps also, quite unwittingly, describes Matthews describing Haslam.'[15] Similarly, Jepson may be describing a parodic version of himself and his methods when he draws attention to Samuel W.'s inquisitiveness and his habit of 'prying and watching'.

Jepson's case-notes continued to show that any interest by Samuel W. in poetry was regarded as being another 'exciting' cause. He recorded on 25 June 1808 that Samuel W. had 'been extremely talkative and fond of writing and reading verses quite in the extreme'.[16] It was mentioned earlier during the discussion of the glass birdcage of patronage that York was the home of Charlotte Richardson, a former domestic servant who had two volumes of poetry published thanks to the highly organised literary philanthropy of Catherine Cappe. Samuel W. seems to have been particularly excited by her poetry, although it is difficult to tell whether this was out of envy or admiration. Perhaps, given his mood-swings, it was both. The case-notes for 1813 record that

> Last 7th day, the 6th of February he went to Charlotte R's about a poem she had written on the Bible Society which he copied and read in the Committee room and ere he had proceeded far, raised his voice in a singing tone – the first manifest symptom of a beginning paroxysm. On first day very flighty, second day worse. Of necessity tied in bed at night – got loose and broke 11 panes in the window of his lodging room. This morning taken into the low back room.[17]

'Flighty' was an imprecise term that was frequently used by Jepson and others in the Regency mad business. One of Samuel's sisters, Elizabeth, was described as being 'at times very flighty arch & assuming'.[18] She had been a governess, a fairly common background for female inmates of asylums, before being admitted to the Retreat (a playwright or novelist might allow Clare to have a reunion with the governess from Holywell in one of the asylums). If Jepson is to be believed, Elizabeth indulged herself in overstated, theatrical behaviour that would not have been tolerated by her previous employers. The suspicion of poetry surfaces again in the notes on Ann L.: 'for the 3 or 4 yeare peculiar in her habits – very fond of being alone, writing poetry & averse to useful employment'.[19] Women readers were often seen as participating in a dangerous recreation.[20]

The Retreat perpetuated in heightened form the gender inequalities of the period, despite the fact that the Quakers had a reputation for providing sane women with religious and secular opportunities. Male inmates had much better access to the library than their female counterparts, who were expected to play more active parts in the day-to-day domestic arrangements of the institution. While men could decide whether they wanted to engage in light tasks such as basket-making and gardening, most of the women were involved in the daily round of washing and cleaning: 'a *few* of the men assist in the garden and house work; and a *large* proportion of the women are employed in various domestic offices, and in sewing and knitting'.[21] Clare worked in the garden at High Beach, returning to one of his previous occupations, but almost certainly did not have to do the dishes and laundry. Jane Aaron, writing about Mary Lamb's confinements in private madhouses after stabbing her mother to death in a particularly brutal attack in 1796, observes that the management of female lunatics corresponded particularly closely with 'the socially approved models for all female behaviour'.[22] The asylums more generally reproduced rather than retreated from what were regarded as social norms. Male employees were usually paid more than female ones.

As has been seen, Clare knew Charles Lamb, who had himself spent a short time in a private madhouse in London, and was aware of this family history. Brother and sister lived together thanks to the relative leniency of the laws on criminal insanity at the time of the murder, although more or less every year Mary had to be sent away to a madhouse for a short period when she became violent again. Clare's language may have been violent and he may have assumed the identities of pugnacious Regency pugilists such as Jack Randall but, within the asylum world particularly at the beginning of his confinement, he was not classified as a violent inmate. Allen makes a point of emphasising this. He describes Clare in 1840 as 'looking very well' and says that 'his mind is not worse'.[23] He tells Cyrus Redding that there is no need for Clare to remain in the asylum. In asylum-speak, Clare was a melancholic rather than a maniac.[24] This begs some questions about what he was doing there in the first place.

It may be that domestic violence holds at least part of the answer, even though this was a taboo subject at the time on which evidence is necessarily sketchy. Taylor, accompanied by a medical man, visited Clare in December 1836 and found him sitting in a corner talking to himself. Taylor declared that 'his mind is sadly enfeebled' and that his wife was no longer able to control him, adding that 'he is very violent, I dare say, occasionally'.[25] When Bishop Marsh visited him earlier on, he had been locked out of the house. He certainly came to subject his wife to the psychological violence of telling her to her face that he was really married to somebody called Mary Joyce, who had been a childhood sweetheart. According to his version, Mary's family considered itself to be a cut or two above the poverty-stricken Clares and put a stop to the relationship. Mary becomes a social aspiration as well as more romantic one. Once again, Clare failed to fulfil great expectations. Like some of the male Romantic poets, he could probably be a domestic monster at times even though he appears to have been an affectionate father. Barleycorn may not have always been the most welcome of guests at home.

It is important nevertheless to try to retain some sort of difficult distinction between Clare's literary and social selves. As Simon Kövesi argues, in addressing a lot of his writing to somebody other than his partner Clare was doing no more than following a very old literary tradition indeed. As Byron playfully puts it in *Don Juan*: 'Think you, if Laura had been Petrarch's wife / He would have written sonnets all his life?' (*B*, p. 489). Addressing poems to Mary Joyce does not, by itself, provide any proof at all of delusion.[26] Yet, as evidenced by letters and his account of his escape from High Beach, Clare carried this idea from his literary world into his social and domestic one. This again is not necessarily proof of delusion. It does however suggest extreme nastiness and spitefulness towards a woman who had had to put up with his mood-swings, Eliza Emmerson's intriguing little teases, his laddism and much else besides. Obsessed with Mary, to whom he thinks that he is married, he does not recognise Patty when she comes to rescue him at the end of his walk from Essex. He thinks that she is 'either drunk or mad' (*BH*, p. 264).[27] There were no visits home, even though these could have been a possibility during the confinement at Northampton. Clare tells his wife, probably in 1842, that she 'can claim me away from this place as your husband' (*LJC*, p. 645), but this does not happen. He writes again in 1848: 'You might come & fetch me away for I think I have been here long enough' (*LJC*, p. 657). He tells one of his sons the following year that 'I have been here Nine Years or Nearly & want to come Home very much' (*LJC*, p. 665). Even a classified maniac like Samuel W. with a record of violence was given more freedom of movement during what were taken to be lucid intervals. Perhaps as always class comes into this: richer inmates whatever their condition simply had more mobility as they had in society at large. Perhaps Patty Clare had just had enough of being told outright that she was second best. It is to be hoped that new biographical evidence may become available about her role (and that of the Vicar of Helpston) in the committal to Northampton, which has always been shrouded in a certain amount of mystery as has the committal to High Beach. If Patty Clare did indeed collude in some way in her husband's confinement, then there is an interesting reversal of roles. The patriarchal pattern was for literary men (William Thackeray and Edward Bulwer Lytton) to pack their wives off to asylums, or else more generally, as will be seen, to get them to question their sanity (Carlyle).

It appears that it was Taylor who took the decision to have Clare confined at High Beach without consulting the Emmersons. They found out about what had happened only some months later and got the name of the asylum wrong.[28] Taylor was Matthew Allen's publisher and clearly believed in the propaganda for moral management. He had, it will be remembered, suffered a breakdown and a period of deliriousness himself, and probably felt that he was acting in Clare's best interests. The idea seems to have been for Clare to spend a relatively short time in the asylum and then return home: the Regency equivalent of a rest cure at a health-farm, or at least this is how the propaganda might have put it. At the beginning of June 1837 a letter from Taylor was delivered to Clare by hand. It contained seven pounds. Although this was the regular payment of a half-yearly dividend, Clare was being provided with some pocket money for the journey. He is told that the bearer of the letter 'will bring you up to Town, & take every care of you on the road'.[29] This was a very different journey from the one that he had undertaken in 1820 in the witty company of Octavius Gilchrist. John Lucas puts it very well when he describes this first journey as uncannily anticipating the one taken by Pip in *Great Expectations*: 'as Dickens's protagonist expects his journey to be a kind of rite of passage, transforming him from the identity of "common labouring boy" to that of gentleman, so Clare must have felt that his arrival in London would mean that he could shed his identity of village labourer and emerge as Poet'.[30] Although as seen Clare was initially disorientated by travelling by coach, he appears to have been in high spirits. He wrote a poem about one of the barmaids at a coaching inn (*EP*, 2, pp. 372–3). Pip and Clare were, however, only just beginning to read some of the confusing riddles in the fame game. When Clare arrived in London in 1837 he was on his way to an asylum rather than to fame and fortune. The difference between these two trips captures, in heightened form, the essence of his literary life. Clare's first surviving letter, to Henson in 1818, exclaims 'how great are my Expectations!' (*LJC*, p. 3). He nevertheless goes on to compare himself with Chatterton, which anticipates how precarious these expectations might turn out to be.

An inmate of the Retreat, Edwin R., eventually published a volume of poetry entitled *Madness, or the Maniac's Hall* (1841). In the Retreat however his writing, like that of Samuel W. and Ann L., was seen as being a danger-signal: 'high, flighty & frolicsome – The complaint is evidently hereditary on the paternal side; ... There had been no weakness of mind & no singularity – though rashly enthusiastic & a writer of verses.'[31] Another inmate, Charles Lloyd, was a published author, known to Southey, De Quincey and the other Lakers, when he entered the Retreat in 1816. Clare, himself a prolific and often accomplished writer of sonnets, admired Lloyd's sonnets. Jepson's notes on him are particularly disparaging: 'has had the advantage of a learned education & early discovered a genious [sic] for poetry but always show'd an unwillingness to apply to any business & posn., a child [who] has been permitted to pursue his own inclination.'[32] This inmate did a bolt and turned up one night at De Quincey's cottage with Jepson's men in hot pursuit. The opium-eater was used to strange nocturnal visitors, although mostly of the imaginary variety. Lloyd complained that in the asylum 'a man of great muscular power' had had specific instructions to 'knock him down' everytime he raised a particular subject.[33] De Quincey sympathises with him and sends him on his way, fortunately without the lethal dose of opium that he apparently gave to one of his other visitors, a passing Malay, according to *Confessions*.

The Quaker attitude towards poetry was not entirely negative. *The Annual Monitor* usually contained poems on religious subjects. The Quaker poet Bernard Barton, who stuck with his day job as a bank clerk after being advised to do so by Byron, contributed reasonably regularly to the *London Magazine*. Attention has been paid recently to another Quaker writer, Isabella Lickbarrow, who was closer to the uneducated tradition both of whose sisters spent time in the Lancaster Lunatic Asylum. Thomas Clarkson's *A Portraiture of Quakerism* (1806) was a sympathetic account of the sect that sought to make its practices seem less foreign to outsiders. It draws attention to the importance of Quakers, with their well-established American connections, in the campaigns for the abolition of the slave trade. There are explanations as to why gambling, dancing and going to the theatre were strictly forbidden to members. The reading of fiction is also seen as a dangerous activity because it encourages 'enthusiastic flights of the fancy, which to sober persons have the appearance of a temporary derangement'.[34]

William Tuke's grandson, Samuel, gave the methods employed at the Retreat considerable publicity through his *Description of the Retreat* (1813). He ranks along with More and Cappe, Taylor and Radstock, Southey and Byron, Carlyle and W.J. Fox, as one of great exponents of public relations in this period. Although he quotes from John Milton and William Cowper (both writers with whom Clare was very familiar), he nevertheless shares Jepson's view that it was dangerous for the inmates themselves to get too close to poetry. The library at the Retreat concentrated on what was defined as useful knowledge. This meant that those inmates who were behaving well were allowed to read history and biography, as well as religious and moral writings. They were also, however, permitted more occasionally to use the subscription libraries in York, although Tuke's own suspicions about these institutions probably meant that visits were very carefully supervised indeed. He believed that 'every rational, not to say serious, person would consider them as calculated to produce the most mischievous effects'.[35] The case-notes on Mary R. show that the kind of fiction supplied by these libraries (Romance, Gothic and Historical) was regarded as having the power to undermine discipline at the Retreat: 'much addicted to novel and romance reading, and ... appears to have cultivated her imagination too much and her judgement too little'.[36] Literature is seen once again as a dangerous addiction. Tuke took it as read that 'the works of imagination are generally, for obvious reasons, to be avoided' by those who were not in remission.[37]

The system of moral management, with its profit and loss account of rewards and punishments, was applied to writing as well as to all other features of life at the Retreat:

> The means of writing are ... sometimes obliged to be withheld from the patient, as it would only produce continual essays on his peculiar

notions; and serve to fix his errors more completely in his mind. Such patients are, however, *occasionally* indulged, as it is found to give them temporary satisfaction; and to make them more easily led into similar engagements.[38]

Samuel Tuke prints in a footnote, for the curiosity of his readers, one of the fruits of this occasional indulgence, an 'Address to Melancholy' written by somebody labouring 'under a considerable degree of active mania'.[39] Perhaps Samuel W. actually got into print after all: good on him.

Those in charge of Regency asylums sought to minimise the opportunities available to inmates to write as this was considered to encourage the great sin of flightiness. Inmates were also not allowed to talk in any detail about their hopes and fears in case this confirmed allegedly irrational perceptions: whether large men with rippling muscles were specifically employed to knock this sort of nonsense out of them is another matter. Samuel W.'s 'scraps of poetry' were therefore usually viewed by his keepers with extreme suspicion. He has to be watched closely, or very narrowly in asylum-speak. The poems were seen as constituting neither useful labour nor useful knowledge. They were useful only in that they provided others with a signal that he was about to take another flight back into madness.

Samuel W. does not, however, seem to have been at all put off by this official disapproval of his activities and may indeed have actually been spurred on by it. He enjoyed perplexing Jepson, in the same way that Matthews relished winding up Haslam and Anne Matthewman worried her keepers by being brazen and lustive. He was apparently 'much agitated' by some poems that he read in 1818.[40] The following year Jepson was very alarmed to spy him 'promoting a new publication, getting pieces in verse printed and making presents of them to his various of his friends'.[41] This was, probably, a scene that was very self-consciously staged to annoy the Superintendent. Poetry, almost regardless of its content, could perform subversive functions within early asylum culture. Clare's distribution of copies of Byron to some of those working at High Beach can be seen as part of a contest with the authorities. Given Byron's reputation, it was a particularly provocative move.

Although difficult to date precisely, there was a gradual change of attitude towards poetry and other forms of creativity within asylum culture during the earlier Victorian period. The Murray Royal Institution for the Insane at Perth first produced its own literary magazine, *Excelsior*, in 1857. Other asylums followed suit, so that by 1866 *The Social Science Review* could carry a long review of such publications entitled 'The Literature of the Insane'. It contains a brief mention of Clare, which emphasises the delicacy and pathos of his asylum writings (5, 1866, pp. 235–49, p. 244). More generally, a number of asylums in the 1840s and 1850s allowed inmates to perform in plays, charades and fancy dress balls. Although such events were carefully supervised, they encouraged the very flights of imagination that those in charge of Regency asylums had sought so hard to curb. There were mixed dances during the winter months at Northampton and single-sex ones at Lincoln (local children were imported to dance with the male inmates, which would cause shock-waves today but provides another reminder of the way in which inmates themselves were treated as children). Dickens wrote an account in 1852 of a mixed dance held at St. Luke's Hospital. Richard Dadd, who served over forty years for the criminal insanity of murdering his father, painted a drop-cloth for the theatre at Broadmoor in 1873, in addition to producing his own work. Medical men became more interested in relationships between creativity and insanity. Thomas Macaulay had stated in 1825 that 'perhaps no person can be a poet, or can even enjoy poetry, without a certain unsoundness of mind'. Earlier Byron had claimed that all poets were very 'near' to madness.[42] Lamb, who arguably knew what he was talking about, argued the opposite in 'Sanity of True Genius' (1826). Macaulay's remarks were reprinted in *The American Journal of Insanity* in 1849 (5, pp. 377–8). Four years earlier the same journal carried a long article by Pliny Earle, the physician to the Bloomingdale Asylum for the Insane in New York, entitled 'The Poetry of Insanity', which dealt with the literary aspirations of some of his patients in a reasonably sympathetic way (1, pp. 193–224).

The shift in attitudes towards poetry in particular and creativity more generally in asylum culture was taking place while Clare himself was an inmate. He began his life sentence under a moral management regime based on that employed at the Retreat. He seems to have written relatively little early on at High Beach. As a result of his friendship with William Knight, the house steward at Northampton, his writing received more encouragement there. Knight nevertheless moved to the Birmingham Asylum in 1850, which meant that Clare had more years to serve without a close ally. His eccentric friend Thomas Inskip, who paid a three-day visit in 1847, had died in 1849. If looked at completely unhistorically, it could be argued that an asylum had some benefits for a writer such as Clare and an artist such as Dadd. Such a romanticised, sentimental view would be mistaken. For starters, asylums were often infernally noisy places, day and night. Bertha Rochester's laugh echoes around Thornfield, a menacing but also thrilling sound for Jane, and there is just one of her.[43] Although extreme hostility towards poetry was gradually replaced by more encouraging attitudes, the asylum world remained one that was fundamentally based around suspicion. Even an inmate's appearance of calm and lucidity had to be treated very cautiously as it could just be a cunning theatrical trick to lull superintendents into a false sense of security. The inmates in their turn suspiciously watched their suspicious watchers, looking for opportunities to stage performances that either mimicked authority or contested it more openly. Samuel W.'s 'scraps of poetry' were important weapons in this daily battle, as were Clare's pugilistic performances and some of his poetic ones.

Prying and watching

Samuel Tuke's *Description* created good publicity for the methods employed at the Retreat. Madness had become a very topical subject since the first Regency Crisis of 1788/89, when it looked as though the mad king, George III, would have to be replaced by his eldest son. This eventually happened at the end of the second Regency Crisis of 1810/11 and the time between these two major constitutional crises was frequently punctuated with further alarms about George's mental health.[44] More publicity was given to madness as a result of the fact that two alleged lunatics, Margaret Nicholson and James Hadfield, had tried assassinate the king (in 1787 and 1800 respectively), which intensified debates about the nature of criminal insanity. This led to changes in the law, which explains why Mary Lamb was treated more leniently than Dadd for a similar crime.[45] Tuke's *Description*, which emphasised that the insane could be cared for in humane ways, provided reassurances for all those who were still concerned about the king's condition. Clare's comment in 1820 that he would be loyal even to a mad king, made to reassure Radstock and then Bishop Marsh of his political correctness, needs setting in this context: 'if the King of England was a madman I shoud love him as a brother of the soil in preference to a foreigner who be as she be shows little interest or feeling for England' (*LJC*, p. 110). The foreigner is Queen Caroline, for whom he had a particular dislike. He appears to have been in a minority in his locality, where there was much support for her (although Earl Fitzwilliam declined an invitation from Caroline to support her in the House of Lords). A related reason for the success of Tuke's book was that it was not a scientific treatise but, rather, an account that was accessible to readers without any specialist knowledge. Although the Tuke family had to employ medical men, their version of moral management was grounded in a belief that concerned and compassionate citizens had major parts to play in the care and cure of the insane. Such good citizens, unlike many medical men, were not tainted through previous association with the more traditional forms of physical restraint and coercion employed in madhouses.

Madness was also topical in the sense that, in the more private sphere, most families had come into contact with it according to the definitions of the time. It is difficult to find gentry and aristocratic families where this was not the case: Austen's brother George, Medora Leigh's sister Augusta and Lady Caroline Lamb's son Augustus were all seen as being mentally deficient. This list could easily be extended. The villagers who claimed that Clare would end up as an idiot in a workhouse were almost certainly drawing on personal experience. Alleged madness was in the family as well as being out there in the newspapers and magazines: Lady Byron set about diagnosing her husband as a result of reading an article in the *Medical Journal*. Madness was everywhere, and yet given the stigma that moral management did not succeed in removing, nowhere. It was, at one and the same time, both highly visible and yet also invisible.

The favourable reception of the *Description* underpinned the hostile questioning of Haslam and others by members of the *Select Committee on Madhouses in England* (1814/15). William Tuke claimed that chains and other traditional implements for restraint were not used at the Retreat even on the most violent inmates. Anxious to affirm that compassionate citizens could and should be entrusted with moral management, he concluded his evidence by also claiming that 'very little medicine is used' at the Retreat (1814/15, 4, pp. 134–5). Although the Retreat prided itself on being innovative, it was in fact putting into practice ideas that had been advanced earlier by, for instance, William Battie's *A Treatise on Madness* (1758), which declared that 'management did much more than medicine'.[46]

The success of the *Description* turned the Retreat into a very public, theatrical experiment. The book notes how 'professional persons, or those peculiarly interested in the subject' had always been encouraged 'to visit *every part* of the establishment'. Those who were about to open their own asylums in Britain and elsewhere frequently took up residence in York so that they could have a sustained period of prying and watching. The Retreat provided the model for asylums in America, such as the Maclean Asylum in Massachusetts, as well as for ones throughout Europe. Samuel Tuke is quick, perhaps too quick, to reassure his readers that 'patients are never exhibited to gratify the curiosity of visitors'.[47] The Retreat may not have been like eighteenth-century Bedlam where spectators paid to mingle on stage with the insane and talk (and sometimes act) dirty with them, but it still exhibited inmates to a more discerning clientele. The American traveller Louis Simond claimed that only those from low social classes were on display when he visited: 'the lowest only of the patients are allowed to be seen; for the Quakers recognise in practice some inequalities of rank.'[48] In addition to showing off his own asylum, Tuke was often invited to visit others, going for instance to inspect Northampton in 1839 shortly after it had opened.

Sidney Smith suggests in his favourable review of the *Description* for the *Edinburgh Review* that one of the reasons for the success of the Retreat was that a 'mad Quaker belongs to a small and rich sect'.[49] Clare made a distinction between Primitive Quakers, whom he admired, and the more prosperous sort, whom he despised. When Samuel W. was admitted in 1803 he paid a guinea a week 'exclusive of wages & board of servant'. A different arrangement was entered into in 1817 when it was agreed that he would pay a hundred pounds a year.[50] Other inmates, unaccompanied by servants and not expecting their own sitting-rooms, usually paid much less. There were provisions for those who could not pay for themselves, provided that their Quaker meeting subscribed to the Retreat. Those who either paid the reduced rate, or had it paid for them, were regarded as short-term inmates who were expected to be cured within a year or so. Perhaps the most damning critique of moral management is that, behind all the public relations about compassion and philanthropic concern, it still operated a 'trade in lunacy' that did not differ that markedly from the practices of other private madhouses.[51]

Samuel Tuke's excellent public relations, together with the topicality of madness more generally, increased the number of visitors to the Retreat. Although the Visitors' Book does not always reveal the exact size of particular parties, the entries for 1816 suggest that somewhere in the region of 250 official visitors came to inspect this embodiment of moral management.[52] Samuel W., one of the richer inmates, may not have been exhibited as much as some others and yet the constant procession of visitors must still have increased his sense of living in a world of prying and watching. He nevertheless appears to have looked upon visitors as potential allies since they at least might take him seriously as a writer. The impending visit of the Russian Royal Family in

1814 found him 'earnestly and anxiously employed about copying some papers respecting the Emperor of Russia'.[53] The Emperor was a tourist in Clare's England. In addition to inspecting an asylum, he also watched some boxing matches in London organised by Gentleman John Jackson.

Some of Tuke's more private statements reveal features of the government of the Retreat that the *Description* itself prefers to ignore. He advocates in a letter written in 1814 the need for 'as complete a system of espionage as possible', going on to recommend that one particular member of staff should become a 'sort of head spy'.[54] Although Tuke and the French medical man, Philippe Pinel, are sometimes rather lazily bracketed together by Foucault and others, there were in fact some striking differences between their approaches. Pinel did not ignore an inmate's delusions, but often staged elaborate theatrical performances to reveal them to be false. His approach was much more interventionist than the one used at the Retreat. The asylum provided stages on which both the superintendents and the inmates could act out versions of themselves and their worlds. Rather than concentrating too much on well-known theatrical events such as the dramas staged by the Marquis de Sade at Charenton, it is important to be attuned to the everyday theatricality of asylum life.[55] Clare's own performances as Jack Randall the boxer and Lord Byron will be set in such a context later on.

Despite some of the differences, Pinel nevertheless agreed with Tuke about the need for a sophisticated espionage system. *A Treatise on Insanity*, which was translated into English in 1806, argues that asylums can be prevented from sinking into absolute chaos only by the ceaseless vigilance of the attendants, who are called 'the interior police' and 'the domestic police'.[56] As far as the male inmates were concerned, Jepson filled the role of 'head spy' with his attendants acting as a police force. Moral management was founded on an increasingly sophisticated system of prying and watching, mainly by employees but also by those who just visited asylums. One way for inmates to contest this constant surveillance was to play, and overplay, the part of an inquisitive spy themselves. There is usually much method in what is seen as madness.

Many of Tuke's contemporaries were persuaded that moral management was a more progressive and humane treatment than traditional methods that emphasised the bestial characteristics of the insane. Some modern writers have been much more sceptical about this claim, the most provocative critique being the one advanced by Foucault in

Madness and Civilisation in the 1960s. He seeks to undermine the humanitarian credentials of the Tukes and Pinel by offering dramatic reversals of their seemingly common-sense assumptions. He, like Carlyle before him, refuses to take the Enlightenment at its own evaluation of itself. Instead of following a progressive chronology of a dark age of physical restraint followed by an enlightened period of moral management, he asserts that the mad were in fact better off in earlier societies. This was because they were visible, rather than being confined in asylums, and thus their voices were heard and could be said to be in dialogue with the voices of reason. As Andrew Scull points out, there is a very 'flamboyant romanticism' at work in the way in which Foucault reconstructs the social attitudes and practices of these earlier periods on the basis of very slender evidence.[57]

Flamboyance is indeed fundamental to both the content and form of Foucault's rhetorical assault on moral management. He asserts that before the birth of the asylum the mad were allowed to be, and were allowed to be seen to be, flamboyant and overstated. He applauds the fact that they were exceedingly frolicsome and lustive. They had a stage and an audience for their performances. Spectators may have responded with forms of verbal and physical cruelty but at least, so Foucault argues, they were forced into a response. He contrasts the daylight, or social, existence and visibility of madness in earlier periods with its perpetual night in the asylums: 'but in less than a half-century, it had been sequestered and, in the fortress of confinement, bound to Reason, to the rules of morality and to their monotonous nights.'[58] Madness should provide a licence for truly wild days and nights but, according to this argument, the Tukes systematically sought to bind it back into a monotonous discourse of classification that spoke and wrote about mad people while studiously ignoring what they themselves actually said and wrote. Foucault declares that neither scientific progress nor humanitarian principle 'was responsible for the fact that the mad were gradually isolated, that the monotony of insanity was divided into rudimentary types'.[59] The driving force is held to be a desire to prevent dialogues between unreason and reason which had the potential to undermine society. Madness is therefore denied the very thing which should define it, namely its outrageous, theatrical flamboyance, and becomes just another problem that requires rational classification. For Foucault the greatest crime committed by the Tukes is that they succeeded in making the mad as dull, boring and monotonous as themselves. This is why he chooses, particularly towards the end of the argument, to fashion his own flamboyant rhetoric which flies free from earlier concerns with changing methods of classification and attempts to address, and celebrate, unreason on and in its own terms.

Foucault casts the Tukes as cruel villains in a story, or counter-myth, that is as rhetorically strong as it is empirically weak about how the asylum reduced madness through confinement to silence and invisibility. As suggested, however, confinement itself is a particularly slippery term since Tuke, through a publication which offered readers a guided tour of the Retreat, exhibited inmates despite his pious assurances to the contrary. Some readers visited the asylum in a more literal sense. Inmates were also being watched all the time by a prying superintendent and his police force. They were both confined and displayed in this particular version of the glass birdcage.

Foucault creates the impression that the Tukes had a coherent and systematic plan to replace madness within the monotony of a domestic regime. Perhaps such a grand strategy was in place by the time of the publication of the *Description*. Earlier texts, often in manuscript, suggest that the Tukes had a much more pragmatic approach. It proved extremely difficult in the early days to recruit satisfactory attendants and thus to implement an effective system of espionage. There was a period at Lincoln when the keepers could not keep off drink, eventually being caught smuggling it into the asylum and maybe not just for their own consumption. Grace Poole needs her pot of porter and private bottle of gin to survive at Thornfield. Barleycorn is a queer fellow: he apparently drives some people mad as well as helping to keep others sane. Thomas Prichard was forced to resign from Northampton amid allegations that he was drinking too much. After Clare had escaped from High Beach, he wrote to Allen to try to recover the copies of Byron that he had lent out. Allen was not very helpful or hopeful. He had had to sack three of his staff since Clare's departure because 'they loved talk & dr(i)nk more than work'.[60] This seems like an usually large turnover of staff even by asylum standards, indicating that High Beach had some serious problems while Clare was there. One of Tuke's acquaintances argued that moral management could not succeed in practice unless the attendants themselves were put under surveillance: 'the keeper must himself be kept. If he be not watched and punished, an asylum is likely to be little beyond an alternation of reciprocal violence between the prisoner and the gaoler.'[61]

Samuel W.'s complaints against his keepers were not upheld, largely because Jepson believed that he was disrupting discipline by playing one attendant off against another. Just as Jepson himself operated what he saw as a benign policy of divide and rule, separating violent inmates from the rest, so Samuel W. is accused of implementing his own anarchic version of such a policy by making friends with some attendants while seeking to stigmatise others. When madness spoke or performed in the Retreat, its voice or style was often uncannily similar to those of the supposedly rational authorities. Samuel W. spied upon spies like Jepson. He tried to have a keeper who restrained him put under restraint. Foucault loftily pronounces that forms of dialogue were no longer possible in the asylum. They may have been difficult to orchestrate, and yet both James Tilly Matthews, Samuel W. and, it will be argued, Clare can be seen as trying to engage in highly theatrical dialogues or contests with authority. Similarly, Ann L.'s rejection of useful employment in favour of poetry and Mary R.'s reading of novels in the face of opposition can be seen as deliberately provocative performances, as was Anne Matthewman's flaunting of her sexuality. Foucault misses what may at times have been an unspoken dialogue, but a dialogue nevertheless, because he is, despite all the radical flamboyance, surprisingly elitist. His enemies are published authors such as Pinel and Samuel Tuke. His friends are well-known writers and painters such as the Marquis de Sade and Goya. The elitism means that he is not at all interested in Clare. He is content just to replace one system with another and remains serenely detached from the individual lives of more ordinary asylum inmates. Tuke and his followers may indeed have tried to silence madness, but the evidence indicates that they never completely succeeded in doing so. By assuming so readily that they did, except in the very special cases of famous creative artists, Foucault is in danger of reproducing the very system that he condemns.

Clare felt that his keepers treated him as if he was a prisoner in that most symbolic of *ancien régime* lock-ups, the Bastille. It was hell on earth, or earthhell as he called it. The bad angels reigned supreme. He also likened his experience to both 'Captivity among the Babylonians' (*LJC*, p. 661) and being in the hold of a slave-ship. He did not want some of his sons to visit him because he was convinced that even innocent visitors were being snared and trapped in this prison, even though the bad angels cunningly kept them out of sight (*LJC*, p. 654). Fears of ensnarement and entrapment are common in the stories told by inmates, as has been seen with James Tilly Matthews. All accounts of asylum life supplied by inmates follow those by Clare in drawing attention to the inhumanity of the attendants. Robert Fuller likened his treatment, or rather mistreatment, at the Maclean Asylum to that undertaken by the Spanish Inquisition.[62] Perhaps the most revealing account of life in a moral management lock-up is John Perceval's

A Narrative of the Treatment Experienced by a Gentleman, During a State of Mental Derangement... (1838). He was confined at Dr Fox's asylum, Brislington House, after what appears to have been a religious breakdown (he became convinced that he had to proclaim the Second Coming). Brislington, which was near Bristol, prided itself on being in the vanguard of asylum culture. Opened in 1806, it was purpose-built and claimed in its public relations to take great care in 'preventing persons of rank and quality from an indiscriminate association with those of inferior manners and conditions'. Its attendants apparently maintained a 'constant unobserved surveillance' and intervened only when it was absolutely necessary to do so.[63]

Perceval himself tells a completely different story. He describes Brislington as a '*mad-house*' rather than an asylum and sees himself as having been trapped in 'the net which is spread by the arts and malice of the lunatic doctors'.[64] This is yet another image of ensnarement. Perceval describes being taken to a secret cell for violent inmates hidden away in the kitchen gardens: 'There was a mattrass of straw, and a pillow of straw, both stinking of the cow-yard, on which I was laid. I was then strapped down with a broad strap over my chest, and my right arm was manacled to a chain in the wall. No explanation of any kind was made to me, and I was left alone to my meditations. For myself, I submitted to every thing with passive resignation, and like a child.'[65] Here and at several other points in his story Perceval shows how his treatment was designed to render him childlike. He was being put back in leading strings. Despite the squalor of this punishment cell, he still felt a certain relief at being free from prying and watching. Even towards the end of his period at the madhouse he is unable to bear 'the gaze of a stranger', who might be part of the elaborate and cunning system of surveillance and ensnarement.[66] Perceval also finds his position as a gentleman (his father had been prime minister until murdered by an apparent lunatic) continually threatened and undermined by the jokey familiarity, as well as the brutality, of the attendants. He becomes particularly incensed when he hears them gloating over the Bristol Riots of 1831 (part of the agitation that surrounded the passage of the First Reform Act) and prophesying the destruction of the upper classes. This seems like a dialogue that was meant to be overheard, and can thus be seen as a play that was staged to annoy members of the audience for it.

Anne Digby remarks that asylums like the Retreat had a 'subterranean element of violence' which it is almost impossible for modern historians to recover, particularly as some instances of it were clumsily deleted from the records.[67] Nancy Tomes, writing of the period after the passing of the 1845 Lunatics Act when institutions had to record their methods of coercion, suggests that there must always have been 'clandestine' violence that never found its way into any of the statistical and other returns.[68] An incident that happened at the Retreat in 1834 confirms such an interpretation. Lady visitors had been involved in inspecting the institution on a regular basis since it opened and, from the point of view of the female inmates, might have represented another part of the omnipresent system of prying and watching. One of their reports states that they 'went over the part of the Retreat occupied by Female Patients, with the exception of some forbidden apartments – they have no particular remarks to offer'.[69] There was an immediate attempt by the Committee of Management to deny that 'forbidden apartments' existed and the ladies in question quickly withdrew their statement. The damage had nevertheless already been done, not least by the casual, matter-of-fact tone of the report.

Although 'forbidden apartments' rarely yield up all their secrets to prying and spying historians, the records that were kept show that moral management as actually practised at the Retreat and elsewhere was accompanied by levels of violence that were denied in the public relations statements. Chains as such may not have been used, and Tuke made a great deal of this in his public relations, but there were plenty of other options: straps, belts, manacles, handcuffs, muffs, wrist-straps and hobbles were all employed in the new asylums. There are fairly frequent references to the way in which Samuel W. was 'waistcoated' and more occasional ones to the way in which cold baths, known in the jargon as the 'bath of surprise', were used to try to control him. He was also sometimes locked away, as has been seen, in a 'low back room'.

Violence was one of the unspoken dialogues that permeated asylum culture. Samuel W. fought back with the tenacity of a prize-fighter on occasions: Clare in the shape of Jack Randall and Anne Matthewman would have been proud of him. He developed a powerful enough kick to break an attendant's shin in 1808. Jepson himself was on the sharp end of this kick in 1813. Samuel W. also used metal chamberpots to good effect as weapons in close combat and, as seen, broke eleven window panes on one occasion before he could be restrained. Windows, perhaps for symbolic reasons, were always particularly vulnerable in asylums. John Conolly, who was one of the pioneers of lack of restraint at the Middlesex County Asylum in the 1830s, noted that 'when restraints were first discontinued at Hanwell, the destruction of windows was said to be ruinous'.[70] Apparently lunatics, cunning devils, liked nothing better than the challenge of a heavily fortified asylum.

This is why their equally cunning keepers attempted to disguise as far as possible the nature of the prison. Matthew Allen proudly reported that at High Beach 'the windows are iron resembling wooden frames'.[71] The Venetian blinds at Brislington were made of heavy iron but painted to look more normal. In addition to breaking windows, Samuel W. set fire to rooms and destroyed furniture. He also put up a good fight when Jepson's men apprehended him as he was travelling back to Alton: 'this morning was with great difficulty brought back quite a maniac by Chas. and John Wansborough nearly having bruised and wounded them and damaged five or six chaises on the journey. Samuel W. has also got several bruises in their contests.'[72] To damage one chaise may be regarded as a misfortune, but to set about trying to destroy five or six of them seems like extreme carelessness towards property and therefore propriety. Perhaps this was just the message that Samuel W. wanted this drama to convey to Jepson. Samuel W. eventually lost this contest, but he certainly went down fighting.

One way of challenging Tuke's public relations is to raise questions about the levels of both recorded and 'clandestine' violence that continued to accompany moral management. Foucault is not interested in this essentially empirical approach because, for all his antipathy towards the systems and classifications that he encounters in the works of those who promoted the idea and ideal of the asylum, he too is a builder of systems. He sets out to demythologise Tuke's account by revealing what he takes to be the system behind the system. He is not interested in continuing levels of physical violence because he wants to show that, behind the façades of 'moral management', there was a systematic use of a new kind of torture that was almost exclusively psychological. He claims that the Retreat's supposedly humane system of indulgences and penalties, rewards and punishments, ushered in a world in which madness was forced to come to terms with the 'stifling anguish of responsibility'.[73] In other words, the mad were driven into prying on and watching themselves. They no longer had wild days and nights of irresponsibility because they became willing participants, or actors, in the espionage system that had been created to spy on them. It is a potentially interesting point, even though Foucault himself arrives at it by a questionable route.

Mischievous children

The case-notes on Samuel W. show how moral management theories about responsibility were translated into practice. If he behaved well, then he was rewarded by being given permission to visit his family or else to have some of them to stay with him. If he was behaving like a naughty little boy, then the visits ceased and he was left to reflect upon the error of his ways in the isolation of his sitting-room. If he responded at all violently to this system of rewards and punishments, trying to contest it, then it was time for physical restraint and institutional violence to come into play. He was waistcoated and surprised by early baths. Allen employed a similar system at High Beach. Having different locations, he could move prisoners about according to their behaviour: 'They are moved from one house & from one part to another according to their behaviour.'[74]

The pioneers of moral management believed that inmates had to be treated as children, who had to learn all over again (or perhaps for the very first time) how to behave in what was regarded as a socially responsible manner. This gave superintendents and others unlimited powers to spy on what were seen to be the antics of mischievous children. Mischievous is a term that is frequently used by the House-Surgeon at Lincoln. Tuke claimed that 'there is much analogy between the judicious treatment of children, and that of insane persons'.[75] Allen believed that insanity was often caused by a lack of discipline in childhood, a view that can also be found in many of Jepson's case-notes. According to P.B. Shelley's own probably exaggerated account, his father threatened to send him to a madhouse when he appeared to be out of control as a boy.

This explains why Allen recommends in his *Essay on the Classification of the Insane*, which was published by John Taylor, that an asylum should be run along the lines of a strict nursery:

> It is a species of discipline like that of a nursery; – children commit some fault, and are removed from the objects of their affection as their punishment; and no punishment is greater or more effectual. Some of our circle break out into a passion, or give way to some strong propensity; they are told it won't do, and are removed: they soon promise to behave better, and return.[76]

Allen's paraphrase of one of his own commands, 'they are told it won't do', can be read in different ways and voices. It nevertheless seems to imply a certain resigned boredom on the part of an adult speaker when confronted, yet again, with highly predictable forms of childishly disruptive behaviour. There are times when these troublesome toddlers simply have to be told who is in charge.

Allen made up for his shaky medical qualifications with his charisma. Like other asylum-keepers, he was very plausible. Tennyson, preoccupied by the threat of hereditary madness as one of his brothers was in an asylum, fell under his spell and visited the asylum while Clare was there. There is a potential novel or play here as well. Tennyson was nearly bankrupted as a result of an unwise business venture with Allen.[77] By the early Victorian period asylum culture was actually producing the very neuroses that it claimed to be able to cure. Jane Welsh Carlyle was by no means alone in frequently checking herself for signs of incipient madness, although she may have been more at risk than most given the extreme moods and eccentricities of her husband. The documentation is not sufficient to answer the question of whether Clare was ever mad, and even if it was much fuller this would still be difficult and perhaps impossible to do. The jury probably needs to be sent home, rather than being kept out. Roy Porter suggests that if Clare was mad, and the if here needs to be seen as a big one, then this might eventually have been produced by spending such a long time in asylums. Once again, asylum culture produces the very conditions that it claims to be able to cure. This is a reasonable scenario.[78]

Madness has been seen here primarily as something which is socially constructed. Having said this, Samuel W., James Tilly Matthews and John Perceval were clearly odd birds. What unites them is a desperate desire to be the centre of attention. Samuel W. is a great poet, Matthews is the diplomat who can solve a major war (seen by some historians as being the First World War) and Perceval goes one better and becomes God's diplomat to announce the Second Coming. If there is to be a clinical account, and again the if needs to be a very big one, then it needs to recognise how very much Clare wanted and needed to be at the centre of literary attention. There may have been a division between his shy, solitary and secretive self on the one hand, and his driven, ambitious self on the other. Yet, as will become clearer in the next chapter, he genuinely believed that he could and should have been able to compete successfully with best-selling authors like Byron. His other impersonations included literary superstars such as Shakespeare, Scott and Burns. He was a very literary person, much more so than is sometimes recognised, and any account of his alleged madness, whether historical or clinical, has to recognise this.

The motto of moral management could well have been that madness 'won't do'. First of all because, as Allen suggests, inmates were seen as offending against notions of decorum, respectability and responsibility. Their sexuality was not under wraps. They disrupted the harmony of a family 'circle' with their self-indulgent, childlike passions. Valerie Pedlar rightly emphasises the problem that somebody from Clare's background might have had in fitting in with these essentially bourgeois constructions of the family.[79] Second, because inmates often seemed unwilling to 'do' anything that was defined as being productive and useful. Ann L. was regarded as being 'peculiar' because she preferred being on her own and writing poetry to being engaged in 'useful employment', which meant doing dishes. Ironically, perhaps, the 'head spy' and his police force at the Retreat did all they could to prevent any form of personal retreat, or flight, from the strict moral values of a social circle. This is why Samuel W. could not get the authorities to take his poetry seriously. The reason for devoting some space here to the task of recovering the literary life of a writer like Samuel W. who did not, strictly speaking, have one has been to recover in turn some of the assumptions on which nineteenth-century asylum culture was built. These have not always been fully understood by some of those who write on Clare who have fallen rather too easily for the plausible public relations of moral management.[80] This needs to be resisted not least because, as will be suggested now, this is what Clare himself did, even though there are some poems that seem to praise the opportunities offered for solitude and retirement (in places away from the asylum buildings). An early letter from High Beach praises the care that he is receiving (*LJC*, p. 642). Yet, like other inmates, he also described asylums as hell on earth, a cage glass all round, in which innocent and harmless people were trapped and then spied on by the bad angels. They, like peasant-poets, were rendered childlike. Unlike Perceval and some of the others who wrote about what it was like to be on the receiving end of moral management, Clare did not succeed in escaping from the clutches of the mad doctors for long. Or perhaps he did in his own way by performing the parts of Regency boxers and Lord Byron.

5
A Government Prison where Harmless People are Trapped: Regency Poets and Victorian Asylums

Fight club

Branwell Brontë possibly pitched up in London sometime towards the end of 1835 with the intention of studying art at the Royal Academy. Yet instead he may have frequented the haunts of prizefighters before returning to Haworth to play what was to become his favourite part of the prodigal son. He may have been spotted by an acquaintance at the Castle Tavern in High Holborn. This was owned by Tom Spring, who had been Champion of England before swelling the ranks of old pugs who kept pubs. It had previously been owned by other famous fighters such as Bob Gregson and Tom Belcher. Branwell prided himself on speaking the flash and playful patter of the boxing fraternity, picked up from reading old copies of *Blackwood's* as well as from the sporting press more generally. The first (and indeed second) rule of fight club was not to talk about fight club except in this coded language. Exhibition matches and sparring, with gloves or mufflers, were within the law: Branwell himself belonged for a while to a boxing club in Haworth. Prizefighting itself like duelling was nevertheless illegal, which was an important part of its appeal. The world of the Fancy offered Branwell the opportunity to escape from responsibilities like finding a career into an underworld in which heavy drinking was not just accepted but expected. The drugs were to come later, partly as a result of a copycat reaction to De Quincey's *Confessions*. He created real as well as imaginary infernal worlds.[1]

Boxing had, like Clare's career, been in decline since the mid-1820s. Spring himself had retired in 1824. Magistrates were becoming more zealous in locating and stopping fights which were classified as riotous assemblies. Although the Fancy prided itself on its patriotism, all large crowds were seen as posing a threat, particularly after Peterloo. Boxing became yet another vice to be suppressed. The Thurtell case, which it will be remembered that Reynolds covered in detail for the *London* and Pierce Egan publicised, badly tarnished the image of the fight game. Gentleman John Jackson closed his rooms in Upper Bond Street: he had been gradually withdrawing from the sport before this. The Fives Court, which Clare had visited in 1824 to watch sparring, was demolished relatively soon afterwards. Accusations about rigged fights, known as crosses, were rife. Aristocratic and gentry patrons gradually withdrew their support, which meant that bareknuckle became a more exclusively lower-class sport. Prosperous middle-class supporters, whose role is often neglected in some of the more mythologised accounts that stress alliances between peerage and people, also withdrew. The centre of gravity started to shift from London and Bristol to the Midlands and the North.

Clare's interest in boxing may have begun because his father had been an accomplished amateur wrestler before rheumatism took its toll. His father was a major influence on him: fuelling his interests in folk songs, as well as this passion for boxing. Wrestling is one of the sports represented in 'The Village Minstrel'. Clare notes in his 'Journal' that at the Helpston Feast 'Wrestling and fighting the ploughmans fame is still kept up with the usual determined spirit' (*BH*, p. 236). The dividing lines between wrestling and boxing were somewhat blurred: holds, locks, trips, throws, presses and butts were all permitted in the boxing ring in this period. Some of these rules were changed in 1838.

Clare asked one of his correspondents in 1828 for news of a particular bout, prefacing his request by stating 'I have a sort of taste for the Fancy & my Father too is a most determined Gossip in its affairs' (*LJC*, p. 448). As has been noted, visitors to the asylums commented on the way in which Clare assumed the identities of various famous fighters. Always an avid reader of newspapers when possible, he kept up with developments in the sport. *Drakard's Stamford News* contained good coverage of boxing. One of Clare's impersonations was of Big Ben Caunt, who did not start fighting until 1835. Yet, generally speaking, his heroes came from towards the end of the so-called golden age of Regency fighting, before the rot set in to boxing and his own career. Clare's excessive drinking, laddism and passion for bareknuckle were all part of his identity as a particular kind of Regency male writer. The peasant-poet may have been invented in the earlier eighteenth century, but the particularly campy, kitschy ways in which Clare was constructed and marketed are also part of this specifically Regency identity. He was of his period, and yet it is still important to recognise that like all good writers he was also at times one of its best critics. The celebrations of pugilism need to be read alongside poems that offer critiques of some of the violent sports and customs of this age.

Clare was fascinated by the career of Jack Randall, probably prompted by Reynolds's admiration for this Prime Irish Lad and Nonpareil (loosely translated as simply the best: the term was later applied to Jack Dempsey, who also came from an Irish background). Even in the asylum Clare continued to be influenced by the *London Magazine* and its agendas. Reynolds writes about Randall in *The Fancy* and probably hit the town with him. Egan records that the boxer and a young lawyer who sounds like Reynolds found themselves up before the magistrates after one Sunday spree: another small victory for the Vice Society. Randall and Reynolds had also timed their saturnalia amiss. Although Randall, whom Keats watched fighting Ned Turner in 1818 in a bout that lasted over two hours, had a reputation for being good with both hands, his trademark punch was a lethal left jab aimed just below the ear, going for the jugular. It was his hammer, his finisher, his gravedigger. He remained unbeaten, made a lot of money and retired to the Hole-in-the-Wall pub in Chancery Lane, which became another meeting place for the Fancy. The Fancy had to be the soul of discretion about its mysterious movements. This was all part of the furtive and frolicsome fun. Hazlitt goes to Randall's pub when he wants to find out details of the fight between Bill Neat(e) and Tom Hickman, the Gaslight Man, which he immortalised in his essay 'The Fight' in 1822. Randall had, as Hazlitt knew from bitter experience, a reputation for still being an awkward customer, particularly if he had been at the blue ruin or gin. So Hazlitt is relieved to be able to get the information from somebody else rather than risk another potentially aggressive encounter with the great man himself. When he was fighting Randall was known for bad-mouthing his opponents. This may have been part of his attraction for Clare, whose bad language in the asylum has already been noted. Egan claims that Randall's language would have affronted the Vice Society.[2] It has already been seen that some of Clare's did. Egan also makes the point that Randall was a self-taught fighter, whose gifts came from nature rather than from tuition and nurture. As the same language was often used about peasant-poets (no matter how much they had actually read), this was another point of contact between Clare and Randall.

While still at High Beach, Clare issued 'Jack Randalls Challange To All The World'. Clare/Randall announces that the 'Champion of the Prize Ring Begs Leave To Inform The Sporting World That He Is Ready To Meet Any Customer In The Ring Or On Stage To Fight For The Sum Of £500 Or £1000 Aside'. He is not bothered 'As To Weight Colour Or Country'. All he requires is 'A Customer Who Has Pluck Enough To Come To The Scratch' (*BH*, p. 266).[3] Randall's own challenges usually specified a weight. Another of Clare's favourite fighters was Harry Jones the Sailor Boy, whom he had watched at the Fives Court in 1824. This was the fighter that he was asking for information about in his letter in 1828. He may also have encountered Spring (who had changed his name from Winter presumably to sound both more youthful and aggressive), whose identity he assumes as well at times in the asylum.

Most of Clare's references to boxing endorse the widely held view that the Regency period represented a high point, after which there was a decline. Although substantially correct, the Regency ring should still not be romanticised, despite the fact that most contemporary and later accounts do so. Sir Arthur Conan Doyle's *Rodney Stone* (1896), written at a time of acute anxieties about the physical degeneration of the nation, looks back fondly to a time when men were men, the breed was the breed. They had the right stuff. They were all game and bottom. Conan Doyle was writing at a time when champions were still predominantly white. Later on, nostalgia for the Regency ring takes on a different kind of racial tone when many of the divisions, notably the heavyweight one, were dominated by black fighters. Instead of waiting forlornly for great white hopes to appear and then disappear just as quickly, they could be found by those who needed them back in Regency England as champions.

Boxers were occasionally killed outright during fights: the Prince of Wales stopped attending bouts after one such death at Brighton in 1788. Injuries could be caused by bad falls in an unsprung ring with no ropes or padded corners, as happened here (Regency fighters could not fight off the ropes in the style that was to be perfected by Muhammad Ali). Ned Turner killed Ben Curtis in 1816 at the end of an exceptionally long bout. Pug M'Gee was sent to prison for six months in 1819 for killing Samuel Eades in the ring: the verdict of manslaughter indicating that this was done in hot rather than cool blood. Simon Byrne died in 1833 after his fight with Deaf Burke, another foul-mouthed fighter. Three years earlier he himself had killed another fighter. Pugs were more likely to die, however, early on in their retirement. Randall himself, Jem Belcher (another publican) and Henry or Hen Pearce, known as the Game Chicken, all died in their early thirties. As a general rule, it seems that it was blows to the body, or stomachers, rather than those to the head that did the most lasting damage (stomacher, an item of female clothing, means something very different in Austen's world). There were nevertheless still a number of punch-drunk fighters who had taken too many blows to the head, known as nobbers or facers. The sheer and sustained brutality of these contests made them a gruesome rather than pleasurable rite of passage for some Regency spectators, much like attending public executions. Becoming what is seen as being a real man has always been a pretty horrific experience. The sound of broken ribs and cracked jaws could be deafening. There was usually blood everywhere by the end of a fight, despite the best efforts of the seconds. These were fights to the finish which were stopped only when one of the fighters could no longer stagger to the scratch to take any more punishment. As at duels, doctors were on hand to treat the injured parties. Hickman had to be bled after very surprisingly losing to Neat. (There were accusations that he had thrown the fight, although Hazlitt was probably right to suggest that he just took his opponent too lightly.) Some fighters remained unconscious for a very worryingly long time after a fight. One of Randall's opponents took half an hour to come round after being on the end of that finisher and then was still not in his right mind. Others had to undergo surgery shortly afterwards, for instance to have broken fingers amputated. Dislocated shoulders, usually caused by falls, also had to be put back. A number of fighters were forced into early retirement after going blind in one eye. Jem Belcher, known as the Apollo of the ring, lost one eye playing racquets rather than in a fight but carried on gamely afterwards. He nevertheless lost the come-back fights in which his right hand was damaged beyond use: he fought gamely on with one eye and one hand. The classical body had become the grotesque one.

A popular belief then and thus now is that the sport was cleaned up during the Regency by Gentleman Jackson, one of the few fighters to come from a moderately prosperous background. According to the legend, a third of the peerage took boxing lessons from him. He certainly built bridges between the patrician world of Byron and the plebeian world of the boxers. Egan describes him as the link that keeps the whole chain together. He and Byron organised at least one fight, on Epsom Downs in 1808. Fights often took place at racecourses, because they provided seating. Jackson's name acted as some sort of guarantee that punters would not normally be cheated or gammoned by thrown fights, bent officials and many other forms of sharp practice. He did not bet himself, which meant that he could claim to be impartial. He refereed the fight between Neat and Hickman (collecting a purse for the loser afterwards) and other important ones. He was master of ceremonies at various boxing events. His rooms, where fencing as well as boxing was on offer, had a cachet and respectability that would have been unthinkable a few years before. Byron, who had a good reach for his size, boxed with Jackson, whom he referred to in his letters as Jack, on an almost daily basis when he was in London for instance during the earlier part of 1814. He recalled that back in 1806 he had lost his temper when sparring with one of Jackson's other pupils and had hurt him.[4] Sparring was a way of trying to keep his weight down: like other pin-ups, this was a constant worry for him. He responded well to the physicality of the sport: 'I like energy – even animal energy – of all kinds.'[5] Byron's Don Juan also boxes when he is in London. What was not so widely reported, except by furtive word of mouth among the secret society of the Fancy, was that locations associated with boxing were also convenient covers for other activities. Jackson, for example, used to pimp for fashionable young men about town. He helped when Byron established Caroline Cameron as his mistress in Brompton in 1808. It is possible that the two lovers first met at one of the parties that Jackson laid on for his young gentlemen to meet women. He found them their love-nest and then dismantled it when Byron inevitably wanted to fly away. The 'Emperor of Pugilism' ran a number of errands for Byron: getting him a new swordstick, helping him to get his money back on a dubious pony and paying for some theatre tickets. He also appears to have helped with cures for sexually transmitted diseases.[6] Leigh Hunt first saw Byron taking part in a swimming match which was being umpired by Jackson. Byron had a screen in his London rooms which was decorated with pictures of Regency boxers.

Jackson probably catered for most sexual preferences. He and his fencing master Henry Angelo (who had visited Byron in Cambridge) were both rumoured to be homosexuals, possibly even lovers. They had the perfect front to broker relationships between men since they had made it legitimate and respectable for male bodies of all classes to be on display to each other. One of the important moments in most fights was when the participants stripped off, which was known as buffing. Jackson himself was described by Egan as 'one of the best made men in the kingdom'.[7] Visiting the molly houses, or male brothels, was a very high-risk activity: raids and blackmail were just around the corner. The shadow of the pillory and the gallows hung over them. Gentleman Jackson, with friends in very high as well as in extremely low places, was a much safer bet. He clearly did much to make boxing more respectable, while remaining aware that part of its attraction would always be that it, and the subculture that grew up around it, promised forbidden pleasures. For a few sadists the main pleasure might well have been watching roughnecks beat each other to pulp in an illegal prizefight. For many others, however, it was prizefighting's associations with sexual as well as criminal underworlds, particularly gambling, that was its main lure.

Jackson himself, like his pupil Byron, may be difficult to place sexually and fights themselves were largely homosocial events. The Fancy was predominantly made up of fancy men. Women did occasionally attend, but this was regarded as being unusual enough to provoke comment, as happened in reports of the contest between Spring and Neat in 1823 and the bout between Ned Painter and Tom Oliver in 1820. Prizefighting's illegality nevertheless meant that it rubbed shoulders with prostitution. Boxing pubs, along with certain theatres, were well-known meeting places. Also, unlike Jackson, many fighters were almost as famous for their heterosexual promiscuity out of the ring as they were for their conquests in it. They were sexual athletes. Tom Cribb was one of the many fighters who led a colourful private life. As Byron put it, he was 'a publican, and I fear, a sinner', having left his wife and moved in with his mistress.[8] Becoming a Regency boxer allowed Clare to assert his heterosexuality in a Victorian environment that was designed to render him childlike. Joyce Carol Oates, writing about modern boxing, nevertheless suggests that there may still be moments when the homosocial shades into the homoerotic. Women are banned from training camps so that the concentration on the opponent can be total. The bout itself is a mixture of dance, courtship and coupling. Despite all the glaring and staring before the fight itself, boxers often embrace each other when it is all over. Oates may be overstating the case here, although it is still important to be reminded that Clare's heterosexual take on boxing is not the only one that is available.[9]

Jackson provided an acceptable public face for boxing, even though his own record as a fighter as opposed to a teacher was a controversial one. He fought only three times. He won his first fight, but lost the second (with George the Brewer) after slipping over in a wet ring and breaking his leg. Fights and fighters were often at the mercy of the elements: it could be raining knives and forks, or even snowing. If magistrates had moved the Fancy on and thus delayed the start of proceedings, fights could finish in darkness. Jackson's main claim to fame was for beating Dangerous Dan Mendoza in 1795. Mendoza was small and quick, bobbing and weaving, dancing like a butterfly in the ring. Jackson put a stop to all this by grabbing hold of Mendoza's hair with one hand (no shaven heads in those days) and then pummelling him in the face with the other: it was a variation on a wrestling hold known as the Chancery lock. Some thought that this was an illegal tactic, but Gentleman John was given the benefit of the doubt: Mendoza had his enemies. Jackson spent the rest of his career dining out on this questionable victory: meeting the Prince Regent, visiting heads of state such as the Emperor of Russia and being generally accepted within high society. He and some of his burly mates were put in charge of crowd control at the Coronation in 1821. They had specific instructions to prevent Queen Caroline from crashing the event. Clare would have approved of this role. Prizefighting and the Regency were inseparable.

Clare's passion for boxing, always present but becoming a distinctive feature of the asylum years, is open to a number of overlapping interpretations. As indicated, he was not classified as a violent inmate (or maniac) even though it seems that there were times, particularly later on, when he got into trouble with the authorities at Northampton and had some of his privileges taken away: he liked to be out all day, only returning to the asylum for meals and to go to bed. At times he might have played the theatrical part of a boxer simply for laughs: there was a potentially comic discrepancy between his small, slight frame and the muscular physiques of some of the incredible hulks and bulks such as Caunt, who were his heroes. Having said this, Randall was one of the smaller fighters at about half the weight of the massive Game Chicken, who topped the scales at over twenty stone and packed a lethal left. At other times the performance might have been more genuinely pugnacious, allowing him to square up to both prying keepers and visitors who seemed to be patronising him. Given the strict social stratifications within asylums, he may also have been delivering a message to the richer inmates of the asylum. To be a plebeian Regency boxer when banged up for life in Victorian institutions designed to inculcate bourgeois values was to make a statement, if not necessarily of subversion or out-and-out defiance then at least of difference. Clare criticism has always been attuned to the way in which he creates golden ages and lost Edens: the landscapes of his childhood; the love that may have been possible for a time with Mary Joyce. The criticism has not, however, been attuned as it might have been about the way in which the particular period of the earlier 1820s also becomes a golden age in his more specifically literary life, particularly when viewed from the perspective of Victorian asylums. This was the period when, as indicated, he might still have achieved sustained literary success. He felt very much part of the *London Magazine* coterie and gained pleasure from laddish rambles and sprees around the metropolis, which included going to boxing matches. One of the Londoners, Barry Cornwall, had actually sparred with the Game Chicken himself. Boxing therefore becomes an important and powerful symbol for the world that Clare has lost: the Regency world of Reynolds and Wainewright, De Quincey and Hazlitt, Lamb and Egan that asylum culture with its emphasis on the suppression of vice has helped to destroy. The Fancy, its very name and all it stood for, was in direct opposition to forms of moral management. The patter of the Fancy, as the quotes from it will hopefully suggest, was playful and frolicsome. Many expressions from the Regency ring are still current today suggesting the continuing appeal of this patter: coming up to (the) scratch; first blood; to throw your hat into the ring; to fight your corner, and so on. Many members of the Fancy were sexually lustive. It may also be the case that in electing to play extremely butch, in-your-face characters like prizefighters Clare was trying to answer those who took the Carlylean line that there was something effete and effeminate about poetry: 'It is well known that I am a prize fighter by profession & a man that never feared any body in my life either in the ring or out of it' (*LJC*, p. 648). Real men belong, or want to belong, to a fight club. They are all game and bottom.

Boxing offered Clare ways of reading the riddles of his literary life. Most Regency boxers were trying to blast their way out of the ghetto, generally coming from the most marginalised sections of society. Randall came from the Irish immigrant community in London. Part of his attraction for Cockney Clare might have been that he was a Cockney fighter: pride of old London town. Mendoza, an East End wideboy, describes at the beginning of his autobiography how taunts about Jewishness got him started in the fight game. Continuing prejudices against him probably allowed Jackson to get away with his most ungentlemanly tactics. Other Jewish bruisers included Dutch Sam Elias who gave raging bull performances, perhaps because as mentioned earlier he often turned up to fights very drunk indeed. He also had a reputation for being a bit of a clown and showman in the ring. Randall beat two Jewish fighters, Ugly or Black Borrock and Aby Belasco. Bill Richmond, born in New York, was a black servant to the Duke of Northumberland, before embarking on a reasonably successful career in the ring after beating a Jewish fighter called Fighting Youssop. He helped to perfect defensive techniques. It seems that he may have taught Hazlitt how to box. Sometimes black fighters were known by the name of their master, as happened with Cropley's Black. Richmond trained a number of black boxers including Young Massa Bristow. The names nearly say it all. Descriptions such as the Paddy, the Jew, the Gypsy and the Black (sometimes the Moor with its shades of *Othello*) occurred frequently in the sporting press. Members of the Fancy embodied the prejudices of the period in heightened form. Considerable hostility was directed towards the black American fighter Tom Molineaux, a freed slave from Virginia, particularly on the occasions in 1810 and 1811 when he tried unsuccessfully to wrest the championship away from England's very own Tom Cribb. The first American championship fight was not until 1816. Molineaux, who was seconded by Richmond, was the better fighter but Cribb was given better training because so much was at stake. Marvellous Molineaux, who had his jaw broken in the 1811 bout, was another fighter who died in his thirties. He had a reputation for being a sexual athlete too. Egan, Cobbett and others situated boxing within the patriotic discourses of the time: fighting with fists was open, manly and British, unlike the cuttings and stabbings in the back favoured in Napoleon's effeminate Europe.[10]

Many fighters came from occupations connected with heavy, unskilled manual labour. There were also, very appropriately, a number of butchers. One of them, Peter Crawley, who went on to hold the Championship, was known as Young Rump Steak at the beginning of his career. Another was nicknamed the Knight of the Cleaver. Clare may not have looked much like a boxer but his truly abject poverty at the time of his discovery, highlighted and turned into a selling point by both Gilchrist and Taylor when they launched him, meant that he could still identify with these other marginalised figures. Boxing and poetry both appeared to provide the only possibilities for working-class lads of exchanging rags for riches, or of going instantly from zero to hero, although for every success story, there were many more broken dreams and lives (and in the case of boxing bones). The career patterns were broadly similar. Fighters generally took on fewer bouts than would be the case today and had shorter careers. A brief moment of fickle fame was likely to be followed by a period, long or short depending on just how much damage had actually been done in the ring by all those stomachers, of obscurity. Clare could and did relate to this: perhaps the equivalent of a stomacher in the literary world was a review by Lockhart in *Blackwood's*. James McKusick puts it very nicely when he says: 'the prizefighters provided attractive role models for his own plucky effort to slug his way into poetic immortality.'[11] Clare so desperately wanted to be a champ among writers.

Successful boxers who had reached championship standard might take over pubs, or else give lessons to young rakes in London and elsewhere. They also toured the country giving exhibitions at theatres and fairgrounds. Others had to sell what was left of their muscle by becoming bouncers and minders. Dutch Sam was one of the bruisers hired to sort out the 'old price' riots at Covent Garden in 1809, an event which provides yet another reminder that Regency theatres could be very noisy places. Fighters were employed as well during parliamentary election campaigns to dish out a bit of grievous bodily harm to opponents. They also gave young swells guided tours of the lower depths. The criminal underworld always needed a fresh supply of heavies. There were some opportunities to continue in the fight game. A bout required not just seconds, bottle-holders and those who knew how to repair cuts quickly, but also an army of former bruisers to make sure that the ring was not broken. There was usually an inner ring, in which the fight took place, and an outer one for officials and patrons which provided a barrier against the crowd. Both were kept clear by bruisers wielding whips: it was not just the fighters themselves who got cut and bruised. If the inner ring was broken, then all bets were off (another expression from the Regency ring that is still current). There might be an attempt to do this for instance if unpopular fighters like Mendoza and Molineaux looked like winning against the odds, or just when the spectators themselves were spoiling for a fight. Sometimes the best boxing action was taking place outside the ring rather than in it. There were at the very least usually plenty of sideshows to the main event on which additional bets could be placed. As fights were illegal, spectators who tried to get in for free could not very well be taken to court. More bruisers were therefore needed to demand the entrance money, with menaces if necessary. Pickpockets, dodgy bookmakers and fly-by-night punters sometimes had to be taught a lesson the hard way. The Fancy policed itself, and it did not go in for softly, softly approaches.

Peasant-poets and fighters came from marginalised backgrounds. They were likely to enjoy a short period of fame followed by a rapid return to obscurity. Another similarity between these two careers is the role played by the patron in them. After watching Jones the Sailor Boy, Clare fantasises about being an aristocrat so that he can patronise him. Perhaps, in his mind's eye, he would have been a more sympathetic patron than Radstock had turned out to be. He describes in these comments his passion for the sport as a 'mania' (*AW*, p. 144). Some of those who visited him in the asylums were to give this term allegedly more precise, medical meanings. The big prizefights depended on patronage. Randall's career was made possible by a Colonel Barton. Cribb won his championship fights, as suggested, because his patrons spared no expense over training. A patron would select a likely prospect in much the same way as he might buy a horse. He then had to meet the cost of training his discovery, known in the playful patter as putting him out to nurse (Clare told one of his visitors that the reason he was in the asylum was to be trained up for a fight). The patron might find his boxer a job in his household, much as Clare might have been employed to garden for General Birch Reynardson if he had played his cards right. Richmond wore for a time the livery of the eccentric Lord Camelford (who was killed in a duel). For rakes like the Earl of Barrymore, who lived very dangerously, a pet prizefighter who could be free with his fists was a useful person to have around late at night down in the lower depths of the underworld. He employed Billy or Bully Hooper, known as the Tinman, for a time. Some Regency households employed rhyming butlers and maids, whereas others preferred fighting footmen with flying fists. Like peasant-poets, boxers were often known through their occupational status as has already been seen with Jones the Sailor Boy and Hickman the Gas-light Man. Another similarity was that bruisers, like peasant-poets, were sometimes identified by their locality. Randall beat a fighter known as West Country Dick. If Clare had been a boxer instead of a poet, he might still have been known as the Northamptonshire Peasant. Other possibilities might have included the Northamptonshire Nobber, the Peterborough Pug and the Stamford Slasher.

Patrons usually put up the stake money and so had most to win or lose. The serious money was nevertheless made through bets which were often very heavy, or deep in the slang. Hazlitt estimated that 200,000 pounds was riding on the outcome of the bout between Neat and Hickman, although this seems to be an exaggeration. Most big bets were hedged. Bets were not just on the result itself, but also spread around on things like the first knock-down, the first blood drawn and on just how long a particular fighter could survive. As these could be placed while the fight was in progress, a fighter might be under instructions from his patron to start slowly and pull punches so that longer odds became available. This was in every way a theatre of violence. Peasant-poets were also under instructions from their patrons, in this case as has been seen to pull poetry that was deemed to be unacceptable. The fighters themselves got a share of entrance money and were able to place bets on themselves, and indeed on their opponents, with a bit of care. They tended only to be well rewarded if their patrons were able to pocket the stake money, along with the proceeds of several successful spread bets. It was a risky business at the top end of market: perhaps there was indeed one lottery even more hazardous than literature. The individual patron had a virtual power of life and death, at least until the foundation of Pugilistic Club in 1814 which attempted to regulate the sport, perhaps not as successfully as is generally supposed to be the case in the romanticised accounts. Nobody could afford to love a loser for very long at all. Some patrons were generous to a fault, settling annuities on their men in the same way that Clare was treated by the local grandees. Subscription funds were also established to help a few of those who had fallen on hard times. Other patrons ruthlessly severed all connections with badly beaten, and often wounded, fighters knowingly condemning them to become very sad acts on skid row for a short period. There was after all a plentiful supply of aspiring fighters in the ghettos and butchers' shops of Regency England, just as new peasant-poets could always been found soodling and sauntering into the field of literature with their trifles. Perhaps that old boxing joke, that illiterate fighters signed documents with a cross whereas their patrons used a double cross, has its origins in this period.

Fight club offered Clare a way of acting out some of the riddles of his literary life. Patrons may not have been quite so powerful in literature, but they could still make careers as Radstock proved for a while with Clare. Although there are a number of similarities, a notable difference was that while some fighters became working-class heroes Clare himself (unlike Burns) made relatively little impact amongst his own class. He identifies with marginal figures who thanks to patronage enjoy popularity and then often fade away into obscurity. He is like the boxers and yet not like them because some of them still achieve the ommon fame that eluded him. The performance is therefore a mixture of recognition and wish-fulfilment. Far from being mad, it can be seen as a perfectly coherent way of continuing his obsessive quest for the true meaning of fame and popularity. He is in dialogue with himself at some points, and at other ones the performances become a way of contesting his confinement under Victorian moral management with its bourgeois code of family values. I am a Regency prizefighter called the Northamptonshire Peasant with pluck and bottom who fears nobody, and that includes customers such as the monstrous regiment of Victorian mad-doctors. I am quite prepared to take on all comers.

It has been shown earlier on that peasant-poets rapidly went out of fashion because it was felt that they could not make earnest and sincere contributions to the Condition-of-England question. Artisans were all the rage. More generally, most Regency figures received a very bad press indeed in the early Victorian period. Dickens's Sir Mulberry Hawk, who was a patron of prizefighting as well as a duellist, is just one of a number of unflattering representations. Mr Rochester has to be maimed and then tamed. Anne Brontë produced a detailed and damning diagnosis of a Regency rake in *The Tenant of Wildfell Hall* (1848). Carlyle fulminated against Regency dandies as well as their tailors, valets and flunkies. Clare's England became associated with bucks and bruisers, rouged roués and randy rakes, duellists and the *demimonde*. Dickens frequently contrasts the absurdity of Regency figures like the Bow Street Runners with the efficiency of the new detective police force. He also caricatures the Regency world of dandies (Lord Mutanhed in *Pickwick Papers* (1836–7)) and deportment teachers (Mr Turveydrop in *Bleak House* (1852–3)). *Dombey and Son* (1846–8) contains a rogues' gallery of Regency characters who prey upon Dombey: Major Bagstock, Lord Feenix and the Honourable Mrs Skewton. Although Mrs Skewton is represented as a childish, lisping Regency beauty whose charms have faded, she is still shrewd enough to realise what a catch Domeby is for her daughter, Edith. To be fair, Cousin Feenix, a Regency dandy who lives on not much a year, probably redeems himself by rescuing Edith from France. Sometimes such figures were represented just as old-fashioned figures of fun, at other times as more grotesque and sinister reminders of a permissive past. For many Victorians, writers such as Egan, with his tales of the underworld and the Fancy, and Harriette Wilson, whose scandalous *Memoirs* (1825) partially unveiled the world of the up-market kept mistress, came to define everything that had to be avoided like the plague.[12]

As suggested, Regency prizefighters had a particular significance and resonance for Clare himself helping him to define his literary life as a working-class writer dependent on patronage, to come to some sort of terms with those two impostors called success and failure. Yet his performances also need to be placed in a wider cultural context. While he was playing the parts of Jack Randall and others, Dickens was just one of a number of writers who were mercilessly caricaturing fight club as well as other features of the Regency as being ridiculous and old-fashioned. To prove that nothing about the Regency was sacred any longer, Dickens even had the nerve in *Dombey and Son* to call his joke fighter the Game Chicken. This Chicken props up the bar of the Black Badger, wears an old-fashioned white greatcoat even in hot weather and is a thoroughly disreputable character who is out to take the gullible

Mr Toots for everything he can get. He boasts about his perhaps mythical victory over the Nobby Shropshire One, although is well beaten by the inexperienced Larkey Boy. Toots consults him about romance and other weighty matters, although his advice never runs beyond a threat to double somebody up. Like the other Regency characters/caricatures, he is a fraud and a phoney. Toots, who eventually sees through him, gives him enough money to buy a pub and is thankful to get rid of him. Dickens's unflattering representation was almost enough to drive old members of the Fancy mad. Perhaps it sometimes did just that.

Boxer Byron

Clare did not just play boxers in the asylums. One day he was Shakespeare, the next somebody who spoke 'Nine Languages' (*LJC*, p. 662). His visitors did not seem to realise that such self-fashioning could at times be frolicsome and funny. He spoke no languages (except perhaps for a smattering of French). His favourite parts, however, usually had some connection with Regency England. He impersonated war heroes such as the Duke of Wellington and Admiral Lord Nelson (acting out John Scott's version of patriotism), and claimed to be Queen Victoria's father. Visitors to the asylum (did Clare really want to see most of them?), who have been followed by later writers, have tended to describe what was happening in terms of a disintegration of identity. It may be that the reverse is closer to the mark, with Clare contesting the restraints and constraints of Victorian asylum culture by playing a medley of specifically Regency characters including sometimes himself in order to assert his Regency identity. He did all the voices. As with the parts of some of the boxers, he may have been playing some of these roles for laughs even if his solemn visitors did not always get the joke. Despite or perhaps because of the tight regimens in the asylums, he loosened up a bit. There is for instance a comic discrepancy between Clare, who appears to have been a somewhat shambolic militiaman, and Wellington. Comedy had never been one of Clare's strong suits, but in the bleak new world of the asylums it becomes a more distinctive part of his repertoire. He had often referred to himself and other labourers, usually ironically, as clowns. He became a real clown on the good days. More generally, the voices that did not fit comfortably with his identity as a squeaky clean peasant-poet get released in the asylums. He is paradoxically at last able to become a particular kind of male Regency writer – excessive, bawdy and satirical – when banged up for life in this Victorian world. This was how he survived.

It is Byron who helps Clare to articulate and hang on to his own Regency identity. The film of *Lady Caroline Lamb* (1972) opens with Byron, on his uppers after returning from his Oriental travels, going into the ring with a black boxer to try to raise the price of a meal. He wins because he is prepared to fight dirty.[13] Boxer Byron is incidentally Clare's own description in a manuscript jotting from 1841 in which there is some seemingly obscure wordplay about iron and a box-iron. This may become more intelligible when (once again) the specifically Regency context is recovered by remembering that one of George Cruikshank's representations of Byron is entitled 'The Separation: A Sketch from the Private Life of Lord Iron ... '.[14]

Clare and Byron's relationship had always been a complex one, made up on Clare's part of a mixture of envy and identification. Clare was suspicious of Byron's theatricality, suggesting that the Greek expedition and the feelings that inspired it were primarily about 'effect & applause'.[15] This seems unduly cynical and begrudging. Clare had been cross at Byron's 'sneering' (*LJC*, p. 302) remarks about Bloomfield in *English Bards and Scotch Reviewers*, and was also not best pleased at seeing Cowper being dismissed elsewhere. Although he was quite comfortable with the existence of aristocrats, for instance the local grandees (it was those who aped them whom he attacked), Byron's title still sometimes troubled him.[16]

Gilchrist, Byron and others were involved in a particularly bitter controversy about the merits of Alexander Pope (whose smooth rhymes Clare generally admired). Clare appears on the very fringes of these fierce and often furious debates, which may have cost Gilchrist his life.[17] Literary life in Regency England had as has been seen its darker sides. Clare thinks that this involvement may lead him to be assaulted by Byron in print. He pictures the haughty patrician poet giving him 'a stripe on my shoulders with his cane'. His response is defiant and plebeian: 'if he meddles with me any where I'll thrash him with plenty of fouled mouthd words depend on 't' (*LJC*, p. 123). Byron is being threatened with some literary pugilism from the Jack Randall school, as it will be remembered Lockhart was to be. Clare is probably remembering the moment in the first canto of *Don Juan* when those that do not kiss Byron's 'rod', or subscribe to his literary views, are told that they will have this rod laid on them, by God (*B*, p. 429). Clare never needed to resort to 'fouled mouthd words' since Byron was employing his cane elsewhere. Perhaps he never would have actually done so anyway since he was conscious of the need to mind his language in public to please patrons, publishers and readers, whatever he may have felt more privately. It was only really in the asylum that such caution could be thrown to the winds.

Byron may be an antagonist to be feared, but he was also a figure through whom the riddles of other Regency literary lives could be read. When Clare watched Byron's funeral procession set off for Nottinghamshire in 1824, his own career was very much in the balance. He had failed to live up to early promise, at least so the critics said. He could no longer trade on being a curiosity: the vogue for peasant-poets was almost over anyway. Yet what many believe to be his best work, *The Shepherd's Calendar*, was still in progress, albeit as seen at the whim of Taylor's many other commitments and his own real and imaginary illnesses. He did not know in 1824 that this would not relaunch his career and transform him from a mere spectator in the crowd into somebody who might be adoringly mentioned by other spectators in the same breath as Byron. He had to pretend not to be ambitious so as not to offend his patrons, but was deeply so. Nobody could write as much unless they were. Drury, no fool and ambitious himself, picked up this driven streak almost straightaway. Byron showed how success could be achieved, even if he also exhibited its high price-tag. It is not too fanciful at all to suggest that, in the early stages of Clare's literary life as a published author, he may well have harboured thoughts of being able to emulate Byron. Burns, whom he also impersonated in the asylum, had become a national institution, so why should he not dream on? Clare's essay on popularity, which has already been referred to in passing in relation to Chatterton, shows the depth of his obsession with Byron and the Byronic. This was published in 1825, a year after Byron's death, and shows Clare still trying to read the riddles of that day in London when he had watched the funeral procession set off. Although Clare does not make the connection explicitly, it is implied that there are some similarities between himself and Byron. They both had 'hasty fame', or woke up and found themselves famous. Clare describes in 'Child Harold' how 'Fame blazed upon me like a comets glare' (*LP*, 1, p. 55), and then goes on to acknowledge in the next line how brief his moment of glory was: 'Fame waned & left me like a fallen star.' Differences are also implied rather than stated openly. Unlike the at times timid and diffident Clare, Byron 'took fame by storm by desperate daring he overswept petty control like a rebellious flood or a tempest worked up into madness by the quarrel of the elements'.[18] The essay opens as if it is going range widely over a number of writers: Chatterton, a Scotch poet called Robert Tannahill and others.[19] Yet Byron takes even this essay by storm: Clare is hypnotised by him, just as he was to be in the asylums. How was it ever going to be possible to compete with him? Shakespeare is held to be a much better writer, but even so it is Byron who holds the attention. Byron also takes over parts of a poem written in 1832 that is meant to be about Sir Walter Scott (*LJC*, pp. 596–9). Scott had been persuaded back in 1820 by Captain Sherwill to give Clare a copy of one of his books, but had made a point of not writing anything by way of a personal dedication in it. It was a deliberate snub. Clare is a member of the writers' club and yet he still has to be made acutely aware of his lowly position on the rungs of this birdcage.

Clare first started reading Byron's poetry in 1818. Drury, Gilchrist, Joseph Henderson and Cyrus Redding all gave him copies of Byron at various points. He frequently asked visitors to give him more, but they seem to have rarely obliged. Byron was a prominent subject for discussion in the *London Magazine*, where his popularity could not be denied even if some of his writings such as his dramas were criticised.[20] Because of the importance that Byron assumes in the early asylum years, there is a danger of forgetting that he was just one of a wide range of authors that Clare was reading. Clare's 'Journal' shows him pursuing many of the agendas of the *London Magazine*, reading Shakespeare and other Renaissance writers. This text shows just how literary he was, as does the contents of his library. There are big gaps such as the novel and European literature (although he had read Dante), and yet he was nevertheless very well read in British poetry and drama. He also had, as indicated earlier, some knowledge of classical writings. He told one of his visitors that he preferred Wordsworth to Byron and, despite being hypnotised by Milord, there is often some ambivalence in his reactions to the writing itself. His Byron is not necessarily always the one on the page but, rather, the one who bestrode the literary stage. He nevertheless praised Reynolds's poetry by mentioning it in the same breath as Byron's work. He enjoyed the first two cantos of *Don Juan*, likening their hero to Egan's characters from *Life in London*: 'the Hero seems a fit partner for Tom and Jerry fond of getting into scrapes and always finding means to get out agen for ever in the company of ladys who seem to watch at night for oppertunitys for every thing but saying their prayers' (*BH*, pp. 174–5). The comment is a perceptive one: Egan and Byron are both drawing on some of the same traditions of pantomime, masquerade and burlesque. There were at least thirteen stage versions of the Don Juan story between 1817 and 1825, and many knew *Life in London* through the various stage adaptations of it.[21] Clare's praise for Byron was not however unreserved.

He found the English cantos hard going: 'Don Juans visit to England reads tiresome and one wishes at the end that he had met with another shipwreck on his voyage to have sent him else were' (*BH*, p. 187). He managed to get a look at Leigh Hunt's biographical account of Byron when he visited Boston in 1828. He came to see Byron not just as somebody who had a bit of fun at Bloomfield's expense, but also as a writer who treated the critics with the contempt that they deserved. Byron's cane or rod could be his friend as well as his enemy: an ally while still belonging to a great rival. This may not be a strictly accurate view of Byron who, like many who dish out criticism, was sometimes sensitive about getting it back, but it helps to explain why a neglected and rejected Regency poet in an asylum should come to forge some sort of identity with him.

Although Clare's repertoire of parts in the asylums may seem to be bewildering not to say crazy, there was some method and consistency in what he was doing. He returns time and again to this period in the earlier 1820s when all things seemed possible: when Wainewright cracked the jokes and bottles, Egan was a best-seller, Reynolds went on benders with Randall, Hazlitt wrote about boxing and Byron's *Don Juan* was the scandalous talk of the town. Why and where did it all go so disastrously wrong? Looking back to this time was an act of nostalgia, but it was also an act of interrogation, a process of trying to see whether there were any small victories that could be plucked from the jaws of the dismal defeat of his great expectations represented by his journey to London in 1837 on the way to High Beach. Clare could have been a contender, as they say in boxing jargon, for Byron's mantle but it never happened and never will. Playing raunchy, Regency Byron was a way of telling the mad doctors and visitors, and perhaps some of the bourgeois inmates as well, to get lost. I am in hell, but you too can go to hell. I am a Satanic poet. It was also a way of thinking through this defeat. As noted earlier, Byron was difficult to place sexually but Clare does not seem to use his Byronic impersonations to explore sexual ambiguity, ambivalence and mobility. He often remains aggressively heterosexual. Byron's Don Juan is, as Camille Paglia puts it, 'partly Byron and partly what Byron likes in boys'.[22] There are a number of references to his smooth face. He is 'a most beauteous Boy' (*B*, p. 691).

Wainewright was a convicted criminal fast becoming a drug addict. There were no more pale yellow gloves. Reynolds, the facetious life and soul of any Regency party, was a washed-up drunk, Egan had gone out of fashion and Randall was no longer terrifying the Hazlitts of this world at his pub. Hazlitt himself had died in pain and poverty. Lamb had fallen over once too often. Carlyle, who came to think of Byron as being a sulky dandy who was incredibly overrated, was setting the sincere and ever so earnest social agenda. Of the London gang or family, only the one who seemed the most likely to die first, the opium-eater, was still a paid or sometimes paid writer. Clare, who was not aware of all these developments, still had a lot of thinking to do in the asylums about the meaning of fame and Byron was a figure around whom he could try to understand it better.

As Frances Wilson puts it, 'Byron hypnotised his own generation and dominated the next'.[23] Three biographies were published in 1830 alone, including one by Tom Moore. Imitating and impersonating Byron was not a particularly strange, or mad, thing to be doing, particularly for another male poet. Early nineteenth-century novels are littered with characters who are doing precisely this: Mr Rochester in *Jane Eyre* (1847) as well as perhaps Heathcliff in Emily Brontë's *Wuthering Heights* (1847), with earlier figures like Captain Benwick in Austen's *Persuasion* (1818) dismally failing to make the grade by not even being able to pronounce one of Byron's titles correctly. Byron also haunted the pages of what was known as silver-fork fiction, representations of high society which were very popular then if not much read now. Early nineteenth-century society was also littered with young men from all social classes who cultivated Byronic looks, attitudes and gestures. They either dressed up (Turkish/Albanian costumes) or down (open-necked shirts with big collars) to play the part. Keats affected the more casual of these Byronic looks. Edward Trelawny, the adventurer who attached himself to the Shelleys and to Byron, was a character straight out of Byron's Oriental tales. Bulwer Lytton probably even had an affair with Lady Caroline Lamb, which was one of the only ways left of being in bed with Byron after his death. Like Clare, Lady Caroline wrote her own versions of *Don Juan*. Trelawny also tried to get into bed with Byron by laying siege to Claire Clairmont, whom Byron had discarded before the birth of their daughter. Byron's doctor, John Polidori, may have done the same. The playing of the Byronic Byron went on everywhere, including of course in his own works. It was by no means just confined to asylums. Women readers were expected to be adoring. Austen was having absolutely none of this. She claims to have gone straight back to her sewing after finishing one of Byron's steamier tales, which had apparently sold 10,000 copies in just one day and 25,000 within a month.[24] Clare's first volume sold well enough, although he was clearly nowhere near this league. James Soderholm shows how the women in Byron's life, such as Caroline Lamb (through *Glenarvon* (1816) as well as her versions of *Don Juan*), Lady Byron and Teresa Guiccioli participated very actively through what they themselves wrote in the creation and perpetuation of some of the Byronic myths and legends.[25] The women in Clare's life did not provide him with that kind of publicity.

There may be elements of comedy in Clare's identification with Byron, given the huge social discrepancy between them. Byron was after all the cosmopolitan traveller who spoke several languages and who died as a result of his political beliefs. His *Don Juan*, unlike Clare's poem, ranges across the whole of Europe: Spain, Greece, Turkey, Russia and England. It might have ended in Revolutionary France. It is an epic that is nevertheless always finding ways of returning to, as well as escaping from, Regency England.[26] Byron had been a wandering exile in his Napoleonic coach since 1816 after a particularly messy separation that had shocked a normally unshockable high society. Clare, by contrast, found it very traumatic to move just three or so miles down the road. He also wondered earlier when describing his first trip to London whether he had any right to travel by coach, as seen. He may have indulged in a bit of casual sex when in London in 1824 and seems to have confessed to that tease Eliza Emmerson about a later affair, but maybe this was because he felt that he needed to emulate Byron (or perhaps it was Burns who was the role model here). Becoming Byron in the asylums was a way of coming to terms with differences. There were nevertheless still important similarities. Peer and peasant, public school playboy and one-time ploughboy may have inhabited different social worlds and yet they both became outcasts. They both spent their last years in a form of exile (one of Byron's most famous poems, 'The Prisoner of Chillon', may have struck some chords for the imprisoned Clare). Lady Byron and Lady Caroline Lamb would have claimed that another similarity was that they were both completely mad. And, of course, they were both poets who were driven by a craving for adulation, while still being deeply suspicious of it.

What might have fascinated as well as infuriated Clare about Byron, even though he does not mention it, is that his Lordship staged a great poetic comeback. He left England in 1816 with his reputation in shreds and yet, with *Don Juan*, he made sure that he would not be forgotten. The comeback that Clare hoped to stage with *The Shepherd's Calendar* never happened. Byron bounces back by being able to reinvent himself yet again. The voices of the Augustan wit and of the anguished, guilt-ridden outcast ('The wandering outlaw of his own dark mind',

B, p. 105) are replaced by one that oozes aristocratic confidence, urbanity and facetiousness. As Philip Martin puts it, an 'after-dinner hauteur' tends to dominate *Don Juan*'s usually breezy conversational tone.[27] The conversation, as conversations do, has many different registers but its overall tone is patrician even when it mimics underworld and sporting slang. Byron's earlier publications had generally been expensively priced, aimed at the upper end of the reading public. He now stages his aristocratic self, particularly in the cantos published by John Hunt, before a more popular and plebeian audience. Hunt brought out different editions of Cantos Six to Eight designed to hit different parts of the market. The cheap edition, priced at a shilling in an attempt to undercut pirated editions, probably sold 16,000 copies. The popular edition of Cantos Nine to Eleven probably sold even more copies.[28] It was some comeback. Byron's scandalous reputation, together with the expectations of sex and sauciness set up by the Don Juan legend, meant that this time around he woke up and found himself infamous, at least as far as many of the reviewers were concerned. But who needs good reviews if they are capable of selling on this scale? Meanwhile as seen Clare had to hawk *The Shepherd's Calendar* from door-to-door, and go over to Boston to try to offload a few more copies. No wonder he became obsessed by Byron and the great differences, as well as some of the similarities, between them.

As seen, *The Shepherd's Calendar* is nostalgic in the way in which it catalogues old customs. Byron's poem, set in the later eighteenth century, is also nostalgic for the sexual customs of libertinism which were coming increasingly under attack from earnest Evangelicals and other self-appointed custodians of respectability. He converted, seemingly effortlessly, this nostalgia into yet another Byronic best-selling commodity. Clare's nostalgia, also at times for the later eighteenth century, was an effort for him to produce and made very little impact. Byron, the comeback king, had once again shown Clare how it was possible to play the literary market and realise great expectations. Clare was nevertheless left to contemplate 'the vast shipwreck of my lifes esteems' (*LP*, 1, p. 397), as he put it in perhaps his most famous poem 'I Am'.

Anne Barton describes Clare's 'Don Juan' as being 'as viciously misognystic as any poem in the language'.[29] Although there is strong competition for this very dubious distinction, this may well be the case. To be accepted as a peasant-poet Clare had to accept in turn censorship, brutal by bad cops like Radstock and more sensitive from good cops like Emmerson and Taylor. He also developed forms of self-censorship. Such caution was no longer necessary: nobody was listening anymore. The patrons and readers had come and gone. Dickens, Carlyle and other Victorian writers were poking fun at Regency figures. The real Game Chicken was probably turning slowly in his grave. Peasant-poets, boxers, Bow Street Runners, dandies, duellists and deportment teachers were now very definitely the day before yesterday's people. Although Boxer Byron retained his readership (more so abroad than in Britain), he was still regarded by many Victorians as a dangerous and shocking figure associated with permissiveness and promiscuity.[30] He was still the bad boy of literature, which was part of his attraction for Clare now that he himself no longer had to be a good little boy. Towards the end of his imprisonment at High Beach Clare was not just re-reading Byron, but also as has been seen lending out copies of his works. He was spreading the subversive word. Byron had a following amongst the Chartists often through pirated editions, proving that Clare was right to notice that Byron's appeal to the lower orders was based on the liberal positions he adopted towards politics and religion. In an environment committed to bourgeois family values the patrician poet becomes somebody around whom some form of opposition can be mobilised. Peasant and peer, so different in many respects, form an alliance against the forces of respectability. They are members of the poetic as well as pugilistic Fancy, prepared to take on all comers at any weight who dare to come to the scratch. Let battle commence. The mad doctors will get a damn good thrashing from Clare and a jolly good caning from Byron. If necessary, Byron will get his kit off, buff and use his fists. The Victorian doctors deserve everything that they are going to get from this very odd couple of Regency poets.

The sexual politics of Byron's *Don Juan* are much too complicated to be discussed here in a book about Clare. It may be that all that can be done is to assert this complexity in contrast to the relative simplicity and directness of Clare's poem. It is quite often argued by modern critics that one of the big tricks that Byron is turning in his poem is to upset expectations by allowing the legendary seducer in his version to be passive rather than active, at worst amoral in an immoral world. Things have a habit of just happening to the hero: shipwrecked, sold into slavery, bought by the Sultana, coming under the influence of Catherine the Great 'just now in juicy vigour' (*B*, p. 695) and so on. Julia, Haidee, Catherine herself and the women in the English cantos make a lot of running. Juan is seductive in part because 'he ne'er seem'd anxious to seduce' (*B*, p. 821). He also appears to be capable of good deeds such as rescuing Leila. Although these sort of playful reversals certainly take place, Regency readers were more aware than modern ones that *Don Juan* was also still meant at one and the same time to shock and offend. The courtesan Harriette Wilson curled up one night with the poem. She then wrote to Byron to advise him not to 'make a mere *coarse* old libertine of yourself'.[31] This advice coming from her is playful, and yet many other readers including some of Byron's friends, also felt that this was how he might be perceived. Moyra Haslett explores the way in which the poem is ultimately a celebration, rather than just a comic deflation, of libertine values. She nevertheless still retains the idea that it works on different levels: 'an ambivalent mixture of proofs of "innocence" and sly insinuations of something more "wicked"'.[32] The narrator is often in the privileged position of having 'seen more than I'll say' (*B*, p. 786), affecting to despise gossip and scandal in the very act of promoting them. There are some rude jokes, for instance the explanation for Juan's success in Russia 'but most / He owed to an old woman and his post' (*B*, p. 706). More generally, however, the narrator usually stops just short of such obscenities. Clare is not as successful in imitating this knowing stance, which reveals in the very act of trying to conceal.

Clare had been unable to get earlier satires such as 'The Parish' published in book-form for fear of alarming his patrons. This was a long poem (over 2,000 lines) that clearly involved a lot of effort. Although normally a fast worker, Clare spent some time revising and polishing this particular text. It was a poem in which he had invested a lot of himself, claiming that it was 'begun & finished under the pressure of heavy distress with embittred feelings under a state of anxiety & oppression almost amounting to slavery' (*EP*, 2, p. 698). There has been some debate about whether this voice is heard in the poem itself, or whether it is a more conventional piece of writing. The answer is that both are true. It draws heavily on eighteenth-century models (again illustrating just how literary Clare was) and yet Elaine Feinstein is still quite right to notice that the 'bluntness, and trenchancy of rhythm and vocabulary suggest an angry man'.[33] It seems likely that not getting such substantial pieces published must have led to feelings of extreme frustration and bitterness. How was it ever going to be possible to compete with Byron when you are unable to get some of your best work published? He never had this trouble. Clare told Taylor in 1826 that he still thought that 'The Parish' was 'the best thing in my own mind that I have ever written' (*LJC*, p. 377), which was perhaps a last desperate attempt either to get Taylor to publish it or arrange for somebody else to do so. He was still trying to get it published in book-form (perhaps more accurately as a pamphlet) in 1835.[34]

Part of this frustration seems to lie behind 'Don Juan', which is a much ruder and cruder satire. It is in many ways a thoroughly nasty piece of work riddled, as Barton suggests, with a hatred for women which is deeply disturbing. They are all, no matter what their social position, frisky whores bent on lying and cheating. Clare had once described his poetic muse as being a 'fickle Hussey' (*LJC*, p. 230) and so may be writing about feelings of creative as well as sexual frustration and impotence. He had often been aggressively and unpleasantly macho about writing. When explaining why he is unable to correct grammar, he explodes 'confound the bitch Ill never be her slave' (*LJC*, p. 231). 'The Parish' can be said to be misogynistic in a general sense in that it contains only one woman character (drawn from eighteenth-century satirical writings), yet it does not have this obsession with infidelity. The woman, Miss Peevish Scornful, eventually runs away with a servant to get married. She is just a silly thing who has read too many silly novels (like some of the characters in Austen's juvenilia) and is desperate to get married. She is not a predatory sex-fiend. The poem attacks seducers such as Young Farmer Bigg and Young Headlong Racket within a model that sees them as active and the unnamed women as passive (another aspect of the misogyny perhaps). This in turn is just a part of a much bigger picture in which petty tyrants prey economically as well as sexually upon the poor.

Lynne Pearce, writing about Clare's other Byronic performance in the asylum, 'Child Harold', suggests that reading the asylum manuscript notebooks with their almost endless string of women's names is to enter the mind of a sex-killer.[35] Clare is compiling catalogues again, but not of wild flowers this time. Pearce argues more generally that the writings of this period do not just abuse women, but also that women are being used as little more than objects to gratify, or not, the male writer. The woman reader is also excluded. These are important points. Not enough feminists have written about Clare, perhaps precisely because of these disturbing features of his work. Pearce's 1991 essay is to some extent an autobiographical account. She was one of the very few critics at this time who was applying theoretical models, in this case ones suggested by Mikhail Bakhtin's work, to Clare's poetry in a sustained way. This led to some very productive readings of Clare's resistance to forms of linguistic enclosure. Her essay explains her decision to quit the study of Clare as she is unable to reconcile it with her feminism. She is certainly right to draw attention to the extreme misogyny in some of asylum writings. She nevertheless seems to overlook the lyricism, loss and anguish – the attempt to recover joy – that is also present.

It is in the forest that surrounds the Epping asylum that Clare comes closest to recovering and rediscovering this joy. The poems may reflect the topography of the asylum itself, and yet there is also a literary frame of reference. Clare's forest in 'Child Harold' may be a place of solitude rather than of the confusing exits and entrances to be found in some of Shakespeare's festive comedies, yet it is still a place where he is able to invent and fashion himself. He marries Mary Joyce there. As in Shakespeare, forest-time does not obey the laws of normal time. Clare is able to become Mary's husband there as well as Lord Byron. He is able to time-travel back to the landscapes of childhood. Forest-time does not have to recognise that Byron and others are in fact dead. As Dylan Thomas puts it at the end of 'Fern Hill', poets may be expelled from the freedom of Eden but they can still sing in their chains, attempting to recover joy.

Clare claims in 'Don Juan' to be married to two unfaithful women, fantasises in his terms about having a 'bonny lass' (*LP*, 1, p. 95) in the forest (echoes of 'Crazy Nell' perhaps), throws in a song to somebody who might have been an old flame and then thinks about buying sex with a prostitute. In the world of the poem women are being paid back for their own serial infidelity. There are contexts into which this performance and parade of sexuality can be placed. As suggested, sexuality becomes part of the battleground in asylums on which daily contests take place. To be sexually active, in thought if not in deed, was one way to assert adult as opposed to childlike status. It was also more generally a way of rattling the bars of the birdcage.

'Don Juan' is obscene not just in some of its language, but also in its overall structure of representation. Yet amidst all the filth and fear, disgust and desire, loss and loathing Clare mockingly declares that he will not actually spell out a four-letter word out of feelings of modesty, despite clearly signalling what it is. At one level it is not very subtle. At another level here and throughout it is the role of the poet that is being self-consciously performed as well as his sexuality. This and other stanzas (where Clare is often dropping into Regency slang) may hark back to the way in which Radstock and others bullied him to clean up his act.[36] 'Don Juan' is his belated reply to the Vice Society: now that there are no loitering listeners anymore I am going to talk really dirty. Left in the world alone I can at last say what I really think. The poem can also be seen as a response to his literary life. Although he had to be modest in the sense of minding his language, he also had to be modest in his ambitions as a writer. Peasant-poets had to be mindful of their lowly social place. Well, to hell with that now that I am in hell: I can become a swaggering, cynical and best-selling aristocrat if that is what I want to be. Tomorrow I think that I shall become Jack Randall and challenge all comers. And the next day I might speak a few of the languages that I do not speak...

Clare becomes Byron in 'Don Juan' and yet is also conscious as well of not being him: 'Lord Byron poh – the man wot rites the werses / & is just what he is & nothing more' (*LP*, 1, p. 99). The stanza continues the running battle that Clare has throughout the poem with Matthew Allen. Clare may adopt the identity of Byron but knows that he is still 'caged' in 'Allens madhouse' (*LP*, 1, p. 99). He is both the powerful patrician poet and the powerless peasant one, and switches between these identities. George Maclennan suggests that the self-conscious assumption of the Byronic identity needs to be seen as a 'gambit' rather than proof of delusion.[37] The critique of Allen, described as a 'keeper of state prisons' (*LP*, 1, p. 98), raises a contradiction that is meant to damn moral management: asylums claim to repress sex and yet 'it' is still everywhere:

> Earth hells or b-gg-rsh-ps or what you please
> Where men close prisoners are & women ravished
> I've often seen such dirty sights as these
> I've often seen good money spent & lavished
> To keep bad houses up for docters fees
> & I have known a b-gg-rs tally travers'd
> Till all his good intents begin to falter
> – When death brought in his bill & left the halter
> (*LP*, I, p. 98)

The stanza appears to start with a continuation of the savage critique of Allen before moving on to include the medical profession as a whole. In common with other asylum writers, Clare remains afraid of being trapped and ensared: 'madhouse traps still take me by the collar' (*LP*, 1, p. 92). W.H. Auden celebrated the openness of Byron's style by declaring that he too wanted 'a form that's large enough to swim in / And talk on any subject that I choose' in his *Letter to Lord Byron* (1936).[38] He wanted to be able to move effortlessly from Wellington to Duke Ellington. Clare's subject matter is however unfair imprisonment and so his poem is necessarily much narrower and more claustrophobic than Byron's and later imitations of it.

Besides the running battle with Allen, the poem is also topical in the way in which it savages the Royal Family and leading politicians of the time.[39] Yet, although Clare is being both topical and more forthright than he has been in the past, he is also returning to some of his core values. His is a lone, and lonely and lonesome voice asserting the need for common sense, fair play and honest practice: in a word, rationality. '– I wish for poor men luck – an honest praxis / Cheap food & cloathing – no corn laws or taxes' (*LP*, 1, p. 91). The voice of reason is nevertheless now caged in an asylum. Taking away the obscenities, the poem is doing no more than clinging to the values of the reforming Stamford Press, the *London Magazine* and John Scott.

It is also clinging to the wreckage of a literary life that had promised so much and, in terms of appreciation and popularity, ultimately delivered so little. It adopts, or tries to adopt, the Byronic swagger and defiance, while still being aware that that journey to London and then to High Beach in 1837 represented the beginning of the end. Byron was a hard, perhaps impossible, act to follow. It was as simple and as brutal as that. Boxer Byron was in some respects a nextdoor neighbour, and yet in others he was a creature from a different planet. When Clare's body was brought back to Helpston by train in 1864 (Taylor died in the same year), there were no toffs on the balconies and no groundlings lining the streets. There were no pretty girls sighing at the very mention of his name. According to some accounts, there was absolutely nobody there at all. In death as in life Byron had all the luck. His popularity could drive other poets forward and keep them sane. If him, why not me? It was also just a little bit maddening (perhaps more) to have to come to terms with the fact that the English are always going to love an aristocrat and his cane more than they are a peasant and his fists.

'Don Juan' deconstructs the nature of composition and reception. It also returns to the themes that obsessed Clare throughout his literary life, namely the meaning of fame and how to get a big slice of it. He wishes towards the end of the poem that he could write in a more aristocratic environment:

> I wish I had a quire of foolscap paper
> Hot pressed – & crowpens – how I could endite
> A silver candlestick & green wax taper
> Lord bless me what fine poems I would write
> The very tailors they would read & caper
> & mantua makers would be all delight
> Though laurel wreaths my brows did ne'er environ
> I think myself as great a bard as Byron
>
> (*LP*, 1, p. 100)

Proper paper and quill pens were luxuries only to be dreamed about at the start of Clare's literary career. He had to use any old scrap of paper that was going, sometimes using his hat as a sort of desk when writing outside. The scraps had to be hidden away in the early days so that he did not get ridiculed for his mad ambitions. His mother threw some of them away by mistake. He made his own ink. He thinks that he is 'as great a bard as Byron', although the sense of the stanza is still that he has not been able to realise this because of his poverty. The final stanza urges the reader to give him some money quickly. The poet and the whore are indeed the same: 'buy the book & help to fill my pocket' (*LP*, 1, p. 101). Byron had never been forced to beg like this. In outlining some of the material conditions that he would have liked to have had as a writer, Clare is possibly remembering Julia's letter from the convent to Juan, 'written upon gilt-edged paper / With a neat little crow-quill, rather hard, but new' (*B*, p. 427). Byron also incidentally rhymes paper and taper. Clare becomes Byron in the asylums, while realising at the same time that this can never be the case.

To Peterborough Station

Peterborough is the location of one of the major Clare archives. Edmund Blunden modestly describes how, with beginner's luck, he and Alan Porter stumbled across it in 1919. This led to the publication the following year of *John Clare: Poems Chiefly from Manuscript*. Although editions discussed earlier by Cherry and Symons still have their admirers, this edition nevertheless marks the beginning of the serious study of Clare (a hundred years after the publication of *Poems Descriptive*).[40] Peterborough is also the place to where some of us head on the way to the annual John Clare Festival, held at Helpston at the beginning of July. Students of Clare, at whatever level, will benefit from contact with the John Clare Society. I walked around Helpston three years ago with a photographer from Lincolnshire, who had been inspired by Clare at school because he showed that working-class children could be just as creative as anyone else. She opened my eyes: pointing out, amongst other things, the way in which social control was so visibly mapped onto the village. The prison, the gallows, the state church and a pub called the Exeter Arms (where Clare's body was laid before it was buried) were all within a stone's throw of each other, some casting their shadows on each other. Everyone can learn things from a day spent at Helpston.

A railway station is as good a place as any to finish off a book which has been about making connections. There have been four main stops. The first was to show the importance of the six volumes of letters addressed to Clare, when cross-referenced with other material, to an understanding not just of his own literary life but to the period more generally. They are a mine of information about Regency patronage, publishing and many other things. This has been a book about Clare's literary life as a peasant-poet, which has established wider literary contexts connected with his promotion and reception. It has considered, amongst other things, different methods of publication such as subscription and speculation, forms of literary philanthropy and the politics of reviewing. It has also looked in detail at the relationships between a writer and his publisher and patrons.

The second objective was to relate Clare's literary life to the Regency period. This meant highlighting the importance of the *London Magazine*: its other contributors and its agendas. This in turn meant being able to contextualise Clare's increasing marginality in the earnest early Victorian period, as well as suggesting that some of his performances of Regency characters in the asylums may have been much more coherent than they have generally been seen to be. Some Clare specialists may feel that too much emphasis has been placed here on the *London Magazine*. All I can say is that I found the evidence, much of which I did not know when I embarked on this book, compelling. Clare was a writer who was, and felt himself to be, part of a literary coterie. This therefore has to be a major part of his literary life.

A third objective was to try to understand Clare's literary life by looking in some detail at the careers of a reasonably wide range of other peasant-poets and artisan-poets, identifying similarities and differences. This has not meant that his relationships with better-known writers have been downplayed. There is detailed work on Byron and the *London Magazine* group (De Quincey, Hazlitt, Lamb and the others). Writers such as Carlyle and Dickens probably figure more prominently here than in previous criticism. Similarly, the well-known women writers referred to here (Wollstonecraft, Austen, Edgeworth, Gaskell and Charlotte Brontë) do not feature that often in Clare criticism. There has also been an attempt to recover the influence of a popular, but academically neglected, writer like Egan on Clare. The journalist John Scott's influence has been considered at some length.

The final objective was to recover asylum culture in archival detail and then place Clare's literary life within it. This was because this was, with the important exceptions that have been referenced, one of the gaps particularly sometimes in the kind of criticism which has tended to take the moral managers, as well indeed as some other authority figures, at their own evaluation of themselves.

There is always a potential danger of Clare criticism turning into boys' own stuff. There are a number of ways of resisting this. One of these is to pay some attention to the darker sides of this laddism. The evidence may be sketchy and yet it still seems probable that domestic violence played some part in Clare's confinement in asylums. Another way is not to take Clare's particular version of masculinity as being normal, natural and given. This has been done here by looking at the way in which the Londoners experimented through performance with a range of different masculine identities. The political and legal structures of Regency England remained firmly patriarchical and, as Wollstonecraft suggests, were reproduced in the domestic sphere. To say that different masculine identities were created through performance is not in any way to deny these general propositions. It is, rather, to suggest that laddism is just one part among many. And it is probably true to say that for Clare himself it was probably just one part among many. Some of his poems on nests, for instance, can be read as complicated attempts to ally himself with feminine qualities such as nurturing, which a masculine world can destroy. He was, as has been suggested, of his period while also being one of its best critics.

Another way of guarding against the kind of assumptions that sometimes drift into Clare criticism is to introduce women writers into the argument. Some of the well-known ones have already just been mentioned. The first chapter also considers Ann Yearlsey, Christian Milne, Phillis Wheatley, Mary Saxby, Ann Candler and Charlotte Richardson. Working on Clare involves visiting some places from which women were largely excluded: the *London Magazine* and prizefights. Their absence has nevertheless been noticed and, when necessary, explained. Similarly, it was mentioned that the cult of the manly artisan-poet marginalised working women writers as well as peasant-poets. Samuel W.'s case-notes proved to be the best main source for the work on asylum culture, partly because they are much more detailed than most and partly because he wanted to be taken seriously as a poet. Yet they were read alongside the case-notes of a number of women inmates: Anne Matthewman, as well as some of the women who were dumped in the Retreat at York. One of the things that it was possible to do with the six volumes of letters addressed to Clare was to reconstruct literary philanthropy by women in this period. The contrasting styles of Eliza

Emmerson and Marianne Marsh were examined in more detail than is generally the case in previous criticism. The opening chapter took a reasonably long look at the way in which Catherine Cappe marketed her discovery, and a much briefer one at the better-known story of how Hannah More promoted hers. There is an important book (or dissertation) waiting to be written on literary philanthropy by Regency women which could include as indicated material on Burns and Hogg, as well as, for instance, on the Countess of Loudon's patronage of Janet Little. As mentioned, uneducated writers allowed women from higher social classes to demonstrate often very formidable organisational skills, which did not have that many other outlets. Women patrons helping other women is one story. The usually suppressed sexual relationships between women patrons and male poets is, as I tried to bring out in the discussion of Emmerson, another one. They are both interesting and important stories. We know a lot more now than when I first started working on Clare about previously forgotten women writers and other marginalised figures such as women readers. I still think that there is more to be recovered about how working-class writers allowed women from higher social classes some space to operate and network within literary circles.

The nature of this literary life has meant that it has been possible to do some justice to Clare's prose writings including his letters. The poetry was always going to present more of a problem: he was a prolific writer whose openness often makes short quotation difficult. There are some readings: two very different early poems, 'Hollywell' and 'Crazy Nell'; *The Shepherd's Calendar* from the middle period with a little bit on the nightmare poems; and 'Don Juan' from the asylum period with a little bit on 'Child Harold'. Other poems, or groups of poems, are referred to more briefly, but referred to all the same. Sometimes, as in the case of 'The Parish', the commentary is spread across the argument rather than being located in one place. The book has nevertheless been primarily contextual rather than textual. This means that it suggests a number of starting points which individual readers can follow up. This is perhaps as it should be anyway. The four main themes mentioned above have been dealt with in some detail. Those that have not been, such as the folk tradition, have nevertheless been given sufficient attention for readers to know where to go to next. I regret, as indicated in an endnote, not having room to reconstruct cultural life in Stamford in more detail.

This book, like some of my other ones, has a strong archive base. It is also similar in that I sometimes drop into a colloquial style. It is possible to be serious without being too solemn and there are a number of different ways of writing up archive material. There are many virtues to writing in your own voice and some vices in hiding behind Mandarin masks. Radstock's objections to slang provided an additional incentive to use it occasionally.

As far as his literary life was concerned, Clare can be seen as a victim of the prejudices that prevented him from becoming a professional writer. He was not Lord Byron, nor was ever meant to be. Alternatively he can, and I think should, be seen as a great survivor who followed Bloomfield's advice and just carried on writing. This is why he has become such a writer's writer. He is also a survivor in the sense that, thanks to his editors, his work now attracts far more interest than that of many of the professional writers of his day. He is for instance probably more widely studied now than Southey.

Asylum records can produce different emotions: anger as well as despondency. They can also, at other times, be very uplifting since many of the inmates were survivors just like Clare. This is why I have felt it to be important to weave some of them and their stories into the tapestry of this literary life, just as earlier on I read Clare's own literary life alongside the experiences of other working-class writers. I have also looked in this chapter at the lives of some Regency boxers.

I am aware that some readers may feel that the presence of these other life stories might at times have reduced the space that is devoted exclusively to Clare himself. While recognising this as a possibility even though I am writing literary history rather than pure biography my argument, in contrast, has been that his literary life becomes much more understandable historically through a knowledge of these other stories. Clare specialists may already be familiar with some of these stories, although not I think with some of the stories of the insane. For them, perhaps there have been times when I have been able to re-tell at least some of these stories in a different way, making different connections with Clare's own literary life. My point throughout, however, has been that many other readers will not have this familiarity with this material. I think, as I argued right at the beginning of this journey, that these other readers, some of whom may be relatively new to Clare, need to know these stories in order to understand the ways in which he was discovered, constructed, marketed and received. As also mentioned at the beginning, I have taken construction, marketing and reception to be the key elements of a literary life. I read some of Clare's poetry and prose. I refer to most of the main events in his life. But I have been writing literary history rather than biography or literary criticism.

This has meant that I have tried to set what I have taken to be the key elements of this literary life within the wider cultural contexts of Regency and early Victorian Britain.

As Clare's story has not been the only one that has been told here, it may be appropriate for his own words to be the last words here. 'I Am' was probably written towards the end of 1846, when Clare had been imprisoned at Northampton for nearly five years. Nobody wanted to claim him. He was in his early fifties. The poem, which Thomas Inskip got published in a local newspaper, has been frequently quoted and anthologised. In Britain, it is read a lot on the radio. I am obviously aware that what recent Clare criticism has been trying to do, quite rightly, is to show the range of his work. I still want to end, however, with what has always been seen as one of his great arias. It is a poem that acknowledges the failure of his great expectations. And yet it is a poem: this writer's writer survived hell on earth by never quite accepting that these expectations were over.

I am – yet what I am, none cares or knows;
  My friends forsake me like a memory lost: –
I am the self-consumer of my woes; –
  They rise and vanish in oblivion's host,
Like shadows in love's frenzied stifled throes: –
And yet I am, and live – like vapours tost

Into the nothingness of scorn and noise, –
  Into the living sea of waking dreams,
Where there is neither sense of life or joys,
  But the vast shipwreck of my lifes esteems;
Even the dearest, that I love the best
Are strange – nay, rather stranger than the rest.

I long for scenes, where man hath never trod
  A place where woman never smiled or wept
There to abide with my Creator, God;
  And sleep as I in childhood, sweetly slept,
Untroubling, and untroubled where I lie,
The grass below – above the vaulted sky.

(*LP*, 1, pp. 396–7)

Notes

1 A cage glass all round: dilettante patrons and literary philanthropists

1. EG 2250, fol 132. no date (February 1820?). In addition to the Reynardsons, he also called on a mad-doctor called Willis, whose family had been involved in the treatment of George III.
2. Northampton Public Library: John Clare Collection (NMS), Manuscripts 43. Letter dated 5 February 1820. Drury was keen that Clare should broadcast to other would-be patrons Reynardson's interest in him, EG 2245, fol 35, letter dated 4 February 1820.
3. EG 2245, fol 35, letter dated 5 February 1820.
4. The catalogue is in the Holywell Papers, Lincolnshire Archives, document 176. The introduction to it makes much ado of the picturesque nature of the gardens. For Clare's tastes in art, see Tim Brownlow, *John Clare and the Picturesque Landscape* (Oxford: Clarendon Press, 1983). Clare reflects upon the reputations of contemporary artists in an asylum poem, 'On the Neglect of True Merit' (*LP*, 1, pp. 21–2). He is, once again, thinking about the wreckage of his own career. He also wrote an 'Essay on Landscape'.
5. It appears from an undated extract from a letter to Clare that his patron, Admiral Lord Radstock, was trying organise such a scheme, John Taylor, Literary Correspondence and Family Papers, Derbyshire Record Office, D 1561, 774/1, Bundles of Correspondence: John Clare: Northamptonshire Poet.
6. Ronald Blythe, *Talking About John Clare* (Nottingham: Trent Books, 1999), p. 45. This is a collection of Blythe's Presidential talks to the John Clare Society, which have always been fresh and creative.
7. See EG 2249, fol 295, letter dated 2 August 1835.
8. I consider Jones as well as some of the other writers in this chapter in more detail in 'Poor Relations: Writing in the Working Class 1770–1830', David B. Pirie (ed.), *The Penguin History of Literature: The Romantic Period* (London: Penguin, 1994), pp. 257–88.
9. John Goodridge (ed.), *The Independent Spirit: John Clare and the Self-Taught Tradition* (John Clare Society, 1994), p. 17. This argument is developed in more detail in 'Identity, Authenticity, Class: John Clare and the Mask of Chatterton', *Angelaki*, 1, 2, pp. 131–48. Most Clare scholars find 'self-taught' the most empowering of the various terms available. I have benefited from a number of conversations with Goodridge. See also Bridget Keegan, 'Nostalgic Chatterton: Fictions of Poetic Identity and the Forging of a Self-taught Tradition', Nick Groom (ed.), *Thomas Chatteron and Romantic Culture* (Basingstoke: Macmillan, 1999), pp. 210–27. Clare was inspired to write by Bloomfield and Bloomfield himself had been inspired by Burns, see Robert Bloomfield: Correspondence 1788–1840, British Library Additional Manuscripts 28, 268, fols 35–7, letters dated 15 June and 30 July 1800. The sharing of a forename was an additional bond.

10. J.W. and Anne Tibble, *John Clare: A Life* (London: Michael Joseph, 1972), p. 154.
11. Mark Storey, *Robert Southey: A Life* (Oxford: Oxford University Press, 1997), p. 205. It will be clear from the number of times that I quote from it that I am much indebted to Storey's edition of the letters.
12. See Peter Levi (ed.), *John Clare: Bird Poems* (London: Folio Society, 1980) for an edition of these poems. Levi is one of a number of modern poets who have been fascinated by Clare who is very much a writer's writer.
13. EG 2248, fol 341, letter dated March 1831. This is quoted in Edmund Blunden, *Keats's Publisher: A Memoir of John Taylor 1781–1864* (London: Jonathan Cape, 1936), p. 194, which is one of the studies that readers should consult when making up their minds about Taylor's role. See also EG 2248, fols 378–9, letter dated 19 July 1831 in which Taylor refers to Southey as a 'blind critic'.
14. *Belinda* (London: Everyman, 1993), p. 33. The phrase is one of the chapter-headings in Pierce Egan, *Life in London*... (London: John Camden Hotten, 1870 edn.). Part of my argument throughout is that Egan was a more important influence on Clare than is generally recognised.
15. For more details on Yearsley, see Mary Waldron, *Lactilla, Milkwoman of Clifton: The Life and Writings of Anne Yearsley 1753–1806* (Athens: University of Georgia Press, 1996). See also Donna Landry, *The Muses of Resistance: Labouring-Class Women's Poetry in Britain 1739–1796* (Cambridge: Cambridge University Press, 1990) and Jerome McGann, *The Poetics of Sensibility: A Revolution in Style* (Oxford: Clarendon Press, 1996), Ch. 7. On peasant-poetry more generally, Rayner Unwin, *The Rural Muse: Studies in the Peasant Poetry of England* (London: George Allen and Unwin, 1954) remains a useful reference work even though landmark studies such as the one by Landry have changed the way in which the subject is conceptualised and historicised. For Unwin's discussion of Clare, see pp. 121–42. Yearsley is also discussed perceptively in Tim Burke, 'Anne Yearsley and the Distribution of Genius in Early Romantic Culture', Thomas Woodman (ed.), *Early Romantics: Perspectives in British Poetry from Pope to Wordsworth* (Basingstoke: Macmillan, 1998), pp. 215–30. Burke is one of the editors involved in Goodridge's major project on labouring-class poets for Chatto and Pickering.
16. Charles Cuthbert Southey (ed.), *The Life and Correspondence of Robert Southey* ... (London: Longman et al., 1849), 6, 3, pp. 212–13. The letter is to Ebenezer Elliott, an artisan-poet who will be discussed briefly in Chapter 3.
17. EG 2245, fol 202, Taylor to Clare, letter dated 14 August 1820. EG 2245, fol 356, Emmerson to Clare, letter dated 28 August 1821.
18. Leslie A. Marchand (ed.), *Byron's Letters and Journals: Famous in My Time* (London: John Murray, 1973), 12, 2, p. 132. Blacket was patronised by the Milbanke family. Byron was to marry Annabella Milbanke, with disastrous consequences for both of them.
19. For profiles of the crazy club, see 'Lost Boys and Fallen Angels', *Uncut*, July 2000, pp. 40–60. Mary Shelley watched the funeral procession going up Highgate Hill and Lady Caroline Lamb apparently saw it on the Great North Road, although only discovered what it was afterwards.
20. Saxby is one of the writers considered in R. Gagnier, 'Social Atoms: Working Class Autobiography, Subjectivity and Gender', *Victorian Studies*, 30 (1987), pp. 335–63.

21. Ann Candler, *Poetical Attempts* ... (Ipswich: John Raw, 1803), p. 17.
22. EG 2245, fol 9, letter dated 21 December 1818. Henson was a bankrupt in 1814 so it is not clear just how far he was really in a position to help Clare, see Eric Robinson (ed.), *The Parish: A Satire* (Harmondsworth: Penguin, 1985), p. 13.
23. EG 2245, fol 10, letter dated 24 December 1818.
24. Charlotte Richardson, *Poems Written on Different Occasions* ... (York: T. Wilson & Son, 1806), pp. v and viii. I deal more fully with the relationship between poet and patron in 'The Maid and the Minister's Wife: Literary Philanthropy in Regency York', Isobel Armstrong and Virginia Blain (eds.), *Women's Poetry in the Enlightenment: The Making of a Canon, 1730–1820* (Basingstoke: Macmillan, 1999), pp. 127–41.
25. *Poems Written on Different Occasions*, p. xvii.
26. In a manuscript in the Peterborough Clare Collection, A 46 fol 6.
27. For a recent account of these literary squabbles, see Jeffrey N. Cox, *Poetry and Politics in the Cockney School: Keats, Shelley, Hunt and Their Circle* (Cambridge: Cambridge University Press, 1998). Clare is not acknowledged here as an adopted Cockney.
28. J.W. and Anne Tibble (eds.), *The Prose of John Clare* (London: Routledge & Kegan Paul, 1951), p. 233.
29. For a good account of Keats's radicalism, see Nicholas Roe, *John Keats and the Culture of Dissent* (Oxford: Clarendon Press, 1997).
30. EG 2250, fol 122, undated letter. Definitions of the term peasant-poet are considered by Elizabeth Helsinger, 'John Clare and the Place of the Peasant Poet', *Critical Inquiry*, 13 (1987), pp. 509–31.
31. For an excellent account of trespassing in Clare's life and works, see John Goodridge and Kelsey Thornton, 'John Clare: The Trespasser', Hugh Haughton et al. (eds.), *John Clare in Context* (Cambridge: Cambridge University Press, 1994), pp. 87–129.
32. As quoted in Louis Simpson, *James Hogg: A Critical Study* (Edinburgh: Oliver & Boyd, 1962), p. 80.

2 That man I would have him to be: public relations and peasant poetry

1. The list is printed in *The Times*, 25 April 1821.
2. As quoted in *The Examiner*, 15 April 1821. There is an account of the inquest on 18 February 1821. Additional details from *The Morning Chronicle*, 14 April 1821, and W.M. Parker, 'Trial for the Murder of John Scott', *Blackwood's Magazine*, 245 (April 1939), pp. 502–14.
3. As quoted in Hyder Edward Rollins (ed.), *The Keats Circle: Letters and Papers 1816–1878* (Cambridge, Mass.: Harvard University Press, 1948), 2, 1, p. 37. This collection contains a number of other letters from Hessey to Taylor, e.g. 2, pp. 400–20 and 431–53, which provide details about their early business relationship as well as showing later on some of the difficulties that they had with a temperamental writer like De Quincey.
4. NMS, 43, letter dated 2 January 1820.
5. As quoted in Ralph M. Wardle, *Hazlitt* (Lincoln: University of Nebraska Press, 1971), p. 484. For an exciting account of Hazlitt's writing, see Tom

Paulin, *The Day-Star of Liberty: William Hazlitt's Radical Style* (London: Faber and Faber, 1998). Paulin is also one of the modern poets who has tried to get Clare taken more seriously. See 'John Clare in Babylon', *Minatour: Poetry and the Nation State* (London: Faber and Faber, 1992), pp. 47–55, in which he writes about Clare's Joycean use of language and likens his sense of being in Babylonian captivity in the asylums to that found in contemporary West Indian-British writings. See also 'Strinkling Dropples: John Clare', *Writing to the Moment: Selected Critical Essays 1980–1996* (London: Faber and Faber, 1996), pp. 161–71.

6. For more details on Fitzwilliam's career, see E.A. Smith, *Whig Principles and Party Politics: Earl Fitzwilliam and the Whig Party 1748–1833* (Manchester: Manchester University Press, 1975). Fitzwilliam was a moderate, or Rockingham, Whig (against parliamentary reform) whereas his son, Viscount Milton, who succeeded him, was a more advanced one.
7. Taylor gave Clare a reasonably detailed account of the duel and its background, EG 2250, fols 333–4, letter dated 17 February 1821, and EG 2245, fol 49, letter dated 21 March 1820 (although the correct date is 1821). He also promised to enclose a newspaper account of the inquest. Byron and Scott had had their differences, particularly over Scott's decision to publish poems written just before Byron's exile that were intended for a private audience. But they retained a respect for each other with Byron making a generous anonymous contribution to the subscription fund for Scott's family. For a discussion of the relationship, see Willard Bissell Pope (ed.) *The Diary of Benjamin Robert Haydon* (Cambridge, Mass.: Harvard University Press, 1960), 5, 2, pp. 482–5.
8. For more details see *Drakard's Stamford News*, 16 February, 23 February and 2 March 1821. The assault took place late in the afternoon of 15 February.
9. EG 2248, fol 339, letter dated 18 March 1831. Extracts from 'The Parish' were published in the *Stamford News* on 18 August 1827.
10. These remarks summarise a range of often fragmentary notes in the Peterborough Clare Collection. For example: A42, fol 94 and fol 132; A45, fol 6, fol 31 and fol 37; A46, fol 43; B5, fol 74, fol 87 and fol 91. I understand that the Clarendon editorial team is producing an edition of Clare's political writings which will be useful (since published: P.M.S. Dawson, Eric Robinson and David Powell (eds.), *John Clare A Champion for the Poor: Political Verse and Prose* (Manchester: Carcanet Press, 2000)). Clare's 'Apology for the Poor' and other pieces are reprinted in Eric Robinson and David Powell (eds.), *John Clare* (Oxford: Oxford University Press, 1984), pp. 445–51.
11. The most accessible account is Patrick O'Leary, *Regency Editor: The Life of John Scott* (Aberdeen: Aberdeen University Press, 1983). See also Josephine Bauer, *The London Magazine 1820–29* (Copenhagen: Rosenhilde and Bagger, 1954), pp. 57–80, 92–118 and 177–219, and Jacob Zeitlin, 'The Editor of the *London Magazine*', *Journal of English and Germanic Philology*, 20 (1921), pp. 328–54. I establish contexts for Clare's politics throughout *English Literature in History 1780–1830: Pastoral and Politics* (London: Hutchinsons, 1983). On the importance of common sense see P.M.S. Dawson, 'Clare and the Ideology of "Common Sense"', *John Clare Society Journal*, 16 (1997), pp. 71–8, and 'Common Sense or Radicalism? Some Reflections on Clare's Politics', *Romanticism*, 2 (1996), pp. 81–97. Dawson is particularly good at isolating different positions within both patrician and plebeian radicalism.

12. See *Recollections of a Literary Life*... (London: Richard Bentley, 1852), 3, 1, pp. 181–99. Other women contributors included Sarah Austin and Elizabeth Kent.
13. I deal with dandyism throughout *Jane Austen and Representations of Regency England* (London: Routledge, 1994), esp. pp. 72–83. See also John Harvey, *Men in Black* (London: Reaktion Books, 1997). As both Harvey and I notice, dandies tended to dress down but this does not rule out a more overstated creature like Wainewright. See also Ellen Moers, *The Dandy: Brummell to Beerbohm* (London: Secker & Warburg, 1960), a book which I think more and more was a very long way ahead of its time.
14. This dinner party is excellently reconstructed by my colleague Andrew Motion, *Wainewright the Poisoner* (London: Faber & Faber, 2000), pp. 100–11. I regret only having a chance to read this after most of my own work was completed. Amongst other things, Motion is particularly good at dealing with the ways in which the Londoners were obsessed with crime and criminality. I have tended to concentrate on their often related obsessions with theatre and theatricality. Motion is yet another modern poet who has tried to promote Clare. See 'Watchful Heart: The Poetics and Politics of John Clare', *Times Literary Supplement*, 8 July 1994, pp. 5–6.
15. 'Pen, Pencil and Poison: A Study in Green', Hesketh Pearson (ed.), *Essays by Oscar Wilde* (London: Methuen, 1950), pp. 73–99.
16. J.W. and Anne Tibble (eds.), *The Prose of John Clare*, p. 228.
17. Byron describes himself in *Beppo* as 'A broken Dandy lately on my travels' (*B*, p. 629).
18. In addition to Motion's work, see John Lindsey, *Suburban Gentleman: The Life of Thomas Griffiths Wainewright: Poet, Painter and Poisoner* (London: Rich & Cowan, 1942), and Jonathan Curling, *Janus Weathercock: The Life of Thomas Griffiths Wainewright 1794–1847* (London: Thomas Nelson and Sons, 1938).
19. Lord Ernle, as quoted in Leonidas M. Jones, *The Life of John Hamilton Reynolds* (Hanover: University Press of New England, 1984), p. 292. Although Reynolds's reputation today is as a minor poet and a friend of Keats, his prose contributions to the *London* (particularly the underworld ones) should not be underestimated.
20. *Life in London*..., pp. 351–2. Although the Fives Court is mentioned as one of the places to visit, Egan's young gents do not in fact go there. They do, however, pay a visit to Tom Cribb's pub.
21. For more details, see Motion, *Wainewright the Poisoner*, pp. 173–4.
22. Lamb's concern about the way in which beggars were being swept off the streets was shared by others. See for example J.T. Smith, *Vagabondia; or, Anecdotes of Mendicant Wanderers Through the Streets of London*... (London: British Museum, 1817). I deal with the representation of beggars in the early Victorian period in 'Platform, Performance and Payment in Henry Mayhew's *London Labour and the London Poor*', Kate Campbell (ed.), *Journalism, Literature and Modernity: From Hazlitt to Modernism* (Edinburgh: Edinburgh University Press, 2000), pp. 54–71.
23. Adam Phillips (ed.), *Charles Lamb: Selected Prose* (Harmondsworth: Penguin, 1985), p. 118. Although Lamb is best known for his Elia essays, recent research indicates that he was also writing drama criticism. See Joe Riehl,

'Lamb's Drama Criticism of July 1823: A New Letter and a New Essay', *Wordsworth Circle*, 30 (1999), pp. 59–63. For more details about his relationship with Clare, see Scott McEathron, 'John Clare and Charles Lamb: Friends in the Past', *The Charles Lamb Bulletin* (July 1996), pp. 98–107.

24. *Selected Prose*, p. 157.
25. For more details see Jane Aaron, 'On Needlework: Protest and Contradiction in Mary Lamb's Essay', Anne K. Mellor (ed.), *Romanticism and Feminism* (Bloomington: Indiana University Press, 1988), pp. 167–84.
26. There was also an appendix, *London Magazine*, 6, pp. 512–17.
27. See EG 2246, fol 3, letter dated 23 January 1822.
28. The poem is not attributed to Clare (or Percy Green), perhaps because it went against the pastoral grain with which readers were familiar. There is a prose account of a dream, 'A Remarkable Dream', written in 1832, *BH*, pp. 253–5. There is also an asylum poem, 'Song Last Day' (*LP*, 1, p. 175), which imagines the end of the world.
29. Biographical details here and later on from Grevel Lindop, *The Opium-Eater: The Life of Thomas de Quincey* (London: Weidenfeld, 1981).
30. For an account of Landon's career that suggests that her success was the result of the way in which she reproduced acceptable notions of female beauty and behaviour see Anne K. Mellor, *Romanticism and Gender* (London: Routledge, 1993), pp. 110–23.
31. EG 2248, fol 302, letter dated 21 December 1830.
32. EG 2248, fols 225–6, letter from H.F. Cary dated 13 April 1830. This a reply to Clare's letter, *LJC*, pp. 493–5.
33. See *The Idea of Landscape and the Sense of Place 1730–1840: An Approach to the Poetry of John Clare* (Cambridge: Cambridge University Press, 1972). Barrell's argument is extremely subtle (depending as it sometimes does on Clare's syntax, placing of a verb and precise choice of a word) and therefore difficult to summarise. He argues, amongst other things, that Clare is not always seeking to return to unenclosed landscapes. There is an appendix, pp. 189–215, that deals with the enclosure process in Helpston itself. Enclosure is also an issue that I discuss in the first part of *English Literature in History 1780–1830: Pastoral and Politics*. The best recent account is probably J.M. Neeson, *Commoners: Common Right, Enclosure and Social Change in England* (Cambridge: Cambridge University Press, 1993), which includes a number of references to Clare. Donald A. Low, *That Sunny Dome: A Portrait of Regency Britain* (London: Dent, 1977), shows that this was also a period that saw the continuation of Highland clearances, pp. 71–5. This book, which deserves to be better known, establishes specifically Regency contexts for a range of writers including Clare, pp. 137–40. Low's 1967 Cambridge PhD was on John Scott.
34. Jones, *Life of John Hamilton Reynolds*, p. 212.
35. See EG 2250, fol 132, letter from Drury, no date (February 1820?). Gilchrist wrote for *Drakard's Stamford News* and had been involved in two duels with somebody associated with the more conservative *Stamford Mercury*, which supported the Marquis of Exeter who was often attacked by Drakard's writers. Scott must nevertheless have felt that Gilchrist's name (as a literary person rather than as a controversialist) would benefit Clare since the article that launched the poet is, unlike most others in the magazine, attributed.

36. NMS 44, letter dated 30 November 1819. See also EG 2250, fol 137, letter from Drury, no date (February 1820?), in which Clare is told that there has to be 'regular & extremely settled conduct' if he wants to be a teacher.
37. EG 2245, fol 282, letter dated 9 February 1821. Taylor also warned Clare about the dangers of heavy drinking. See, for example, EG 2245, fols 309–10, letter dated 7 April 1821. Eliza Emmerson also joined in the attempt to sober Clare up. See, for example, EG 2245, fols 397–8, letter dated 21 December 1821. I deal again with Clare's drinking in the next chapter when discussing a Victorian biography. There may be some denial on his part, but perhaps some exaggeration also by those who were promoting him. He lived into old age by the standards of the time (unlike say Branwell Brontë) and was in good physical shape throughout much of the asylum period.
38. NMS 43, letter to Taylor dated 28 August 1819. Taylor uses the same expression in a letter to Clare, EG 2245, fol 62, letter dated 16 March 1820. In another letter to Taylor dated 3 June 1819 Drury writes that with 'careful management' Clare could be a success-story.
39. For an account of Clare's earlier religious beliefs see Mark Minor, 'John Clare and the Methodists: A Reconsideration', *Studies in Romanticism*, 19 (1980), pp. 31–50.
40. For more details of this incident see EG 2246, fol 88, Thomas Bennion to Clare, letter dated 21 July 1822.
41. *The Shepherd's Calendar; with Village Stories and Other Poems* (London: Taylor and Hessey, 1827), p. viii.
42. I deal in more detail with these events in the second part of *English Literature in History 1780–1830: Pastoral and Politics*. One of the best accounts of radicalism in this period is by Iain McCalman, *Radical Underworld: Prophets, Revolutionaries and Pornographers in London, 1795–1840* (Oxford: Clarendon Press, 1993), which also has useful commentary on SSV. I have benefited from conversations with McCalman about the 1820s. David Worrall's *Radical Culture: Discourse, Resistance and Surveillance 1790–1820* (Hemel Hempstead: Harvester Wheatsheaf, 1992) is also recommended. Again, I have benefited from conversations with Worrall.
43. Details and quotations from Charles Pedley, *The History of Newfoundland*... (London: Longman et al., 1868), pp. 175–7. Additional material about Radstock's Governorship from D.W. Prowse, *A History of Newfoundland*... (London: Eyre and Spottiswoode, 1896), pp. 372–4 and pp. 418–19.
44. For Hobhouse's letter advising against publication, see Peter W. Graham (ed.), *Byron's Bulldog: The Letters of John Cam Hobhouse* (Columbus: Ohio State University Press, 1984), pp. 256–61.
45. For the reception of *Don Juan* see Andrew Rutherford (ed.), *Byron: The Critical Heritage* (London: Routledge & Kegan Paul, 1970), pp. 159–205. See also Moyra Haslett, *Byron's Don Juan and the Don Juan Legend* (Oxford: Clarendon Press, 1997), Ch. 2.
46. Marchand (ed.), *Byron's Letter and Journals*, 6, p. 106.
47. See Eric Robinson (ed.), *The Parish*, p. 93, for details of local prosecutions for the crime of playing marbles on a Sunday (notes by David Powell).
48. EG 2247, fol 44, letter dated 11 July 1825. Radstock wanted all his letters returned, whereas earlier Eliza Emmerson had suggested that it was only necessary to destroy some of them.

49. EG 2245, fol 376, letter dated 3 November 1821 (from Eliza Emmerson who is quoting and paraphrasing a letter from Radstock to her). Radstock expected Clare to reply by return to letters from himself and other patrons. Clare is told by one of his corresponents on 25 May 1820 that the Admiral is 'very angry' with him for not answering letters and is thus petulantly refusing to send some books, Peterborough A60, Captain Sherwill to Clare.
50. *John Clare and the Bounds of Circumstance* (Kingston and Montreal: McGill-Queen's University Press, 1987), p. 18.
51. NMS 43, letter to Taylor dated 20 February 1820.
52. *The John Clare Society Journal*, 14 (1995), is devoted to 'Clare and Ecology'. Richard Mabey describes him as a 'naturalist and ecologist of startling originality and relevance', p. 5. Poems that are used as evidence for such claims by critics tend to include 'The Lamentations of Round Oak Waters' and 'The Lament of Swordy Well' (not published in Clare's lifetime). For links between criticism and ecology more generally, see also 'Romanticism and Ecology', *Wordsworth Circle*, 28 (1997).
53. Robinson and Powell (eds.), *John Clare*, p. 149.
54. EG 2245, fol 139, letter dated 6 June 1820.
55. See, for example, a letter from Taylor to his father dated 15 February 1820, John Taylor, Literary Correspondence and Family Papers, Derbyshire Record Office, D 1561, 774/1, Bundles of Correspondence: John Clare: Northamptonshire Poet.
56. For more details, see Philip W. Martin, *Mad Women in Romantic Writing* (Brighton: Harvester Press, 1987).
57. EG 2246, fols 346–7, letter dated 31 May 1824, fols 351–2, letter dated 14 June 1824 and fols 356–7, letter dated 13 July 1824.
58. EG 2249, fol 161, letter dated 31 August 1833. See EG 2249, fol 228, letter dated 16 August 1834 for the publisher's response.
59. EG 2246, fol 134, letter dated 17 December 1822. Emmerson suggested that Clare should put the letters in a 'box securely locked' and bring them down to London next time that he visited so that between them they could decide which ones needed to be destroyed.
60. EG 2245, fol 119, letter dated 11 May 1820.
61. From a letter dated 5 January 1821 in which Taylor anticipates some of Radstock's objections to *The Village Minstrel*, John Taylor, Literary Correspondence and Family Papers, Derbyshire Record Office, D 1561, 774/1, Bundles of Correspondence: John Clare: Northamptonshire Poet.
62. EG 2245, fol 272, letter dated 6 January 1821.
63. For instance this was her advice about 'The Hue and Cry' and 'The Summons'. See EG 2248, fols 395–6, 17 October 1831. I deal with both these poems, which had previously not attracted the attention of Clare scholars, in *English Literature in History 1780–1830: Pastoral and Politics*. See *LJC*, pp. 522–3, for Clare's account of the Swing riots in his locality.
64. EG 2247, fol 213, letter dated 23 September 1826. I discuss letter writing by Regency women in Chapter Two of *Jane Austen and Representations of Regency England*. This particular correspondence is openly flirtatious: 'My very dear Clare' often gets sleepy, late night letters. There are poems on Valentine's day and so on. Having said this, however, Clare is also being drawn into gossiping about topics such as health which formed one of the main subjects

when women in this period wrote to each other. Paradoxically perhaps, as well as being flirted with, he is also being feminised to some extent.

65. EG 2247, fols 126–7, letter dated 10 January 1826.
66. For more details see Bob Heyes, 'Some Friends of John Clare: The Poet and the Scientists', *Romanticism*, 2 (1996), pp. 98–109.
67. EG 2245, fol 186, letter dated 25 July 1820.
68. This point is also emphasised by Merryn and Raymond Williams (eds.), *John Clare: Selected Poetry and Prose* (London: Methuen, 1986), p. 13. Their introduction also contains a detailed account of the construction of the identity of the peasant-poet. This introduction is more attuned to the complexities and contradictions of Clare's literary life than Raymond Williams's work on him in *The Country and the City* (London: Chatto & Windus, 1973), which wants him to be a protest poet pure and simple. I acknowledge Williams's influence elsewhere, in the dedication of one of my Renaissance books to him.
69. For more details see *Hansard*, 5, 14 June 1821, pp. 1160–80 and 7, 7 June 1822, pp. 824–46. Marsh also spoke in the Lords on Catholic Emancipation (emphatically against) and the divorce of Queen Caroline (for, with reservations). Although most of his writings deal with specifically religious controversies, some of them address wider themes. *The History of the Politicks of Great Britain and France*... (London: Stockdale, 1801) lays the blame for the Revolutionary wars firmly on France.
70. I am pleased that this relationship, which has not received the attention that it deserves, will be discussed in more detail than I can offer here by Alan Vardy in his forthcoming study *John Clare: The Making of a Peasant Poet*. Examples of Marianne Marsh's correspondence (sometimes dictated to her companion, Mary Anne Mortlake) include EG 2247, fols 408–12, letter dated 15 February 1828; EG 2248, fols 182–3, letter dated 26(?) October 1829; EG 2248, fols 368–9, letter dated 6(?) July 1831; EG 2249, fol 271, letter dated 24 January 1835; EG 2249, fol 315, letter dated 9 January 1836; EG 2249, fol 353, letter dated 31 December 1836; EG 2250, fol 1, letter dated February 1838 (to Clare's wife); EG 2250, fol 250, n.d. (invitation to dine at the Palace); EG 2250, fol 253, n.d. (invitation to the theatre).
71. See, for example, June Wilson, *Green Shadows: The Life of John Clare* (London: Hodder & Stoughton, 1951), p. 198, which makes good use of the letters addressed to Clare. The story was first circulated, in a more exaggerated form, in a Victorian biography by Frederick Martin that will be discussed in the next chapter.
72. I discuss representations of Jewishness on the Renaissance stage in *Christopher Marlowe* (Basingstoke: Macmillan, 1991), pp. 96–100. Kean was an excessive, heavy-drinking Regency character who was involved in a 'criminal conversation' trial in 1825 as a result of his affair with Charlotte Cox. He thus helped to identify this period with scandal.
73. EG 2248, fols 247–8, letter from Frank Simpson dated 18 July 1830.
74. EG 2250, fol 120, no date.
75. EG 2245, fol 343, letter dated 14 July 1821.
76. EG 2247, fol 65, letter dated 6 September 1825.
77. Although as indicated I do not like the way this issue has been polarised, it has been so I have to present the references like this. Accounts that are

sympathetic towards Taylor's role as editor include Zachary Leader, *Revision and Romantic Authorship* (Oxford: Clarendon Press, 1996) and Tim Chilcott, *A Publisher and His Circle: The Life and Work of John Taylor, Keats's Publisher* (London: Routledge & Kegan Paul, 1972), Ch. 4. I find the commentary in studies by Storey and Barrell, already cited, measured and helpful. The case against Taylor dates back to Eric Robinson and Geoffrey Summerfield, 'Taylor's Editing of *The Shepherd's Calendar*', *Review of English Studies*, 14 (1963), pp. 359–69, which has been elaborated upon (as well as modified) in subsequent publications, most of them already cited. On literary collaborations more generally, see Jack Stillinger, *Multiple Authorship and the Myth of Solitary Genius* (Oxford: Oxford University Press, 1991). His second chapter is a fascinating account of the input that Taylor and other members of the Keats circle had with one of the poems.

78. EG 2245, fol 192, letter from Robert Hankinson dated 29 July 1820. Hankinson had visited Clare the previous day. He went on to become Archdeacon of Norwich.
79. *The Idea of Landscape and the Sense of Place 1730–1840*, p. 141.
80. EG 2247, fol 152, letter dated 4 March 1826.
81. *John Clare and the Bounds of Circumstance*, pp. 125–6.
82. Mark Storey, *The Poetry of John Clare: A Critical Introduction*, p. 95, makes a similar point. His reading is particularly good at showing the literary tradition in which Clare was working, and when he may have been able to transcend it.

3 The importance of being earnest: manly artisans and sincere sages

1. See for example EG 2247, fol 322, Taylor to Clare, no date, and EG 2247, fol 353, letter dated 20 November 1827. There was a downturn in the economy in 1825 which led to banks and other businesses going bust. For some more details see A.A. Watts, *Alaric Watts: A Narrative of His Life* (London: Bentley, 1884), 2, 1, pp. 219–22. A number of publishers besides Taylor and Hessey went out of business (for instance, Hurst, Robinson and Company, Constable and Company).
2. As quoted in John Saville (ed.), *The Life of Thomas Cooper by Himself* (Leicester: Leicester University Press, 1971; facsimile of 1872 edn.), p. 282.
3. *Essays: English and Other Critical Essays* (London: Dent, 1967), 2, 2, p. 165. For a good recent account of Carlyle's social criticism see Michael Levin, *The Condition of England Question: Carlyle, Mill, Engels* (Basingstoke: Macmillan, 1998).
4. *Essays*, p. 199.
5. *Essays*, p. 172.
6. *Past and Present* (London: Dent, 1966), p. 4.
7. *Godfrey Malvern; or the Life of an Author* (London: Thomas Miller, 1842), 2, 1, p. 93.
8. NMS 52, letters dated 20 February 1848 and 14 April 1849. Inskip and Clare shared an admiration for Bloomfield.
9. Charles Kingsley, *Miscellanies* (London: Macmillan and Co., 1863), 2, 1, pp. 357–407, p. 405.

10. *Charles Kingsley: His Letters and Memories of His Life* (London: Kegan Paul, Trench, & Co., 1882), 2, 1, p. 147.
11. See Margaret Farrand Thorp, *Charles Kingsley 1819–1875* (Princeton: Princeton University Press, 1937), pp. 2–3, 5 and 75 for references to Marsh's influence on Kingsley's father. The father had been Rector of Barnack from 1824 to 1830, until in the finest traditions of clerical nepotism the living was given to one of Marsh's son. Barnack is close to Helpston (perhaps allowing Marianne Marsh to combine visits to Clare and her son).
12. *Alton Locke: Tailor and Poet, an Autobiography* (London: Ward, Lock, Bowden & Co., 1892), pp. 114–16.
13. *Alton Locke*, p. 305.
14. Eric Robinson and Geoffrey Summerfield (eds.), *Selected Poems and Prose of John Clare* (London: Oxford University Press, 1967), p. xiv.
15. For Fox's influence, see Isobel Armstrong, *Victorian Poetry: Poetry, Poetics and Politics* (London: Routledge, 1993), Ch. 1. This also contains some commentary on artisan and Chartist poetry, pp. 191–8. There is an intriguing reading of Clare in relation to Matthew Arnold, pp. 219–23, as well as commentary on Samuel Bamford, pp. 222–4.
16. Walter Dexter (ed.), *The Letters of Charles Dickens* (London: Nonesuch Press, 1938), 3, 1, p. 433. *Household Words* did nevertheless carry an article that emphasised Bloomfield's rural virtues, 5, pp. 357–9.
17. Autobiographical Memoir, dated 21 June 1841, Sheffield Public Library, p. 6. Elliott and Clare were influenced by many of the same poets. See J.W. King, *Ebenezer Elliott: A Sketch* (Sheffield: S. Harrison, 1854), p. 14, for similarities in their responses to James Thomson. Spenser and Goldsmith were also shared influences.
18. 'Corn-Law Rhymes', *Essays*, 2, 2, p. 140. Elliott mentions Clare in one of his poems, and Clare was aware of his work through the correspondence of Emmerson, Taylor and Cary.
19. *More Verse and Prose by the Corn Law Rhymer* (London: Charles Fox, 1850), 2, 1, p. 131.
20. 'John Clare, The Northamptonshire Peasant', *Eliza Cook's Journal*, 3, pp. 241–3. It may be significant that Clare should make this brief appearance in a publication edited by a woman who was attuned to the ways in which the cult of the artisan marginalised other writers, particularly women writers (the journal highlighted the exploitation of women servants, governesses, needlewomen and many others). This was incidentally one of the journals that Clare may have had access to at Northampton. For more details on artisan writings, see Brian Maidment (ed.), *The Poorhouse Fugitives: Self-taught Poets and Poetry in Victorian Britain* (Manchester: Carcanet, 1987), pp. 307–9. See also Maidment, 'Essays and Artisans – The Making of Victorian Self-taught Poets', *Literature and History*, 9 (1983), pp. 74–91. Other important studies include Nigel Cross, *The Common Writer: Life in Nineteenth-Century Grub Street* (Cambridge: Cambridge University Press, 1985), Ch. 4, 'The Labouring Muse: Working-Class Writers and Middle-Class Culture'; Louis James, *Fiction for the Working Man 1830–50: A Study of the Literature Produced for the Working Classes in Early Victorian England* (London: Penguin, 1974), Appendix One, 'Some Minor Poets and

Poetry', pp. 201–11; Anne Janowitz, *Lyric and Labour in the Romantic Tradition* (Cambridge: Cambridge University Press, 1998); Martha Vicinus, *The Industrial Muse: A Study of Nineteenth Century British Working-Class Literature* (London: Croom Helm, 1974), Ch. 4, 'Literature as a Vocation: The Self-Educated Poets'. Cross also deals with the Royal Literary Fund from which, it will be remembered, Clare received a grant.

21. Madeline House and Graham Storey (eds.), *The Letters of Charles Dickens* (Oxford: Clarendon Press, 1969), Pilgrim Edition, 2, p. 428. For the text of Overs's letter to Dickens about Carlyle, see Sheila M. Smith, 'John Overs to Charles Dickens: A Working Man's Letter and its Implications', *Victorian Studies*, 18 (1974), pp. 195–217. Her study of social-problem writings, *The Other Nation: The Poor in English Novels of the 1840s and 1850s* (Oxford: Clarendon Press, 1980), considers some of the writers discussed in this chapter and includes work on representations of rural poverty in Kingsley and Disraeli, pp. 97–122.
22. For Coleridge's drinking, and that of his son Hartley, see Anya Taylor, *Bacchus in Romantic England: Writers and Drink 1780–1830* (Basingstoke: Macmillan, 1999), pp. 93–156. There is only a very brief reference to Clare, as a writer of drinking songs. The term Romanticism, and the baggage that comes with it, does Clare no favours.
23. For a more favourable judgement, see Eric Robinson and Geoffrey Summerfield's introduction to a reprint of *The Life of John Clare* (London: Frank Cass, 1964), pp. xiii–xvii.
24. *Rhymes and Recollections of Handloom Weaver* (London: Smith, Elder, 1845 edn.), p. 45. There is a short chapter on Thom in Owen Ashton and Stephen Roberts, *The Victorian Working-Class Writer* (London: Cassell, 1999), pp. 46–57, which suggests how ambitious he was as a writer. The book makes good use of the records of the Royal Literary Fund.
25. Letters and Papers by or Concerning William Thom (1798/9–1848), King's College Library, Aberdeen, Mss. 2304/4.
26. From a letter to David Vedder, another poet, as quoted in Robert Bruce, *William Thom, The Inverurie Poet – A New Look* (Aberdeen, Alex. P. Reid & Son, 1970), p. 91.
27. John Dix (sometimes known as Ross), *Lions Living and Dead* (London: Partridge and Oakley, 1852), p. 165.
28. As quoted in Robert Gittings (ed.), *Recollections of Writers: Charles and Mary Cowden Clarke* (Fontwell: Centaur Press, 1969), p. 273.
29. See *The Northern Star*, 17 August, 24 August, 31 August and 7 September for coverage of the Burns Festival and related issues. There is a long review of Thom's poetry on 14 September. Harney admits on 5 October that the claims on behalf of Burns's daughter may have been exaggerated. He reports on 16 November on a plan to train Sarah Parker, whose poetry was eventually published in book-form in 1846, as a teacher. Thom was later to contribute to the *Star*, for instance an article of 25 April 1846 about Burns's reputation. Harney was the scourge of the aristocracy, but always made an exception in the case of Lord Byron. *The Chartist Circular* was another radical publication that dealt extensively with literary matters.
30. For a discussion of some women poets and autobiographers from the working classes, and their virtual exclusion from an increasingly professionalised

idea of literature, see the second half of Julia Swindells, *Victorian Writing and Working Women: The Other Side of Silence* (Cambridge: Polity, 1985). Writers considered include Mary Barber, Ellen Johnston and Mary Smith. For *The Lowell Offering*, see Benita Eisler (ed.), *The Lowell Offering: Writings by New England Mill Women 1840–1845* (New York: HarperTorchbooks, 1997). Harriet Martineau produced an edition for the British market, *Mind among the Spindles*... (London: Charles Knight, 1844). She had visited the Lowell factory, as had Dickens, who also recorded his experiences, *American Notes and Pictures from Italy* (London: Oxford University Press, 1975), pp. 65–70. As often happened when working-class writers were discovered, there were those who doubted whether the women were in fact the real authors.

31. The Forster Collection ..., Victoria and Albert Museum, Mss. 9 (130 Letters and Notes ... by Douglas William Jerrold), fol 110. Letter dated 20 September 1844.
32. The Diary of Samuel Bamford, 28 February 1858 to 26 December 1861, Manchester Central Library, 4 vols, 1, 24 March 1858. For a considered view of Bamford's politics which rejects the view that he was just a turncoat, see Martin Hewitt, 'Radicalism and the Victorian Working Class: The Case of Samuel Bamford', *Historical Journal*, 34 (1991), pp. 873–92. I did my work on the diary before the publication of Martin Hewitt and Robert Poole (eds.), *The Diaries of Samuel Bamford* (Stroud: Sutton, 2000).
33. As quoted in W.H. Challoner (ed.), *The Autobiography of Samuel Bamford* (London: Frank Cass, 1967), 2, 1, p. 27.
34. As quoted in Challoner (ed.), *Autobiography*, 2, p. 248.
35. Diary, 2, 29 July 1859. Elizabeth Gaskell and Charlotte Brontë were introduced to each other by Kay-Shuttleworth.
36. Diary, 2, 30 July 1859.
37. Diary, 2, from a letter dated 10 August 1859.
38. J.A.V. Chapple and Arthur Pollard (eds.), *The Letters of Mrs. Gaskell* (Manchester: Manchester University Press, 1966), p. 84.
39. Diary, 2, 16 May 1859.
40. *Mary Barton: A Tale of Manchester Life* (London: Penguin, 1985), p. 154.
41. For a short but good account of the way in which John Barton becomes a monster, see Chris Baldick, *In Frankenstein's Shadow: Myth, Monstrosity and Nineteenth-Century Writing* (Oxford: Clarendon Press, 1987), Ch. 4.
42. The English join in Burns night celebrations on 25 January. There is no Clare night.
43. For the Burns manuscript, see Edward Nehls (ed.), *D.H. Lawrence: A Composite Biography* (Madison: University of Wisconsin Press, 1957), 3, 1, pp. 184–95.
44. For an accessible collection of Gothic material from the magazine, see Robert Morrison and Chris Baldick (eds.), *Tales of Terror from Blackwood's Magazine* (Oxford: Oxford University Press, 1995). This includes Hogg's 'The Mysterious Bride', pp. 115–30.
45. *Jasmin: Barber, Poet, Philanthropist* (London: John Murray, 1891), p. 54.
46. For more details, see George Deacon, *John Clare and the Folk Tradition* (London: Sinclair Browne, 1983). The editors of the Clarendon editions are particularly good at identifying folk sources.

47. David Vincent, *Bread, Knowledge and Freedom: A Study of Nineteenth-Century Working Class Autobiography* (London: Methuen, 1982), remains an important study.
48. For more details of Clare's writings on this subject, see Claire Lamont, 'John Clare and the Gipsies', *John Clare Society Journal*, 13 (1994), pp. 19–31, and Anne Janowitz's more theoretically aware account, 'Clare Among the Gypsies', *Wordsworth Circle*, 29, 3, pp. 167–70. See also her 'Wild Outcasts of Society: The Transit of the Gypsies in the Romantic Period', Gerald Maclean et al. (eds.), *The Country and the City Revisited: England and the Politics of Culture 1550–1850* (Cambridge: Cambridge University Press, 1999), pp. 213–30. See *BH*, pp. 83–7 for a prose description of gypsy life.

4 High, flighty and frolicsome: mad poets and moral managers

1. The phrase comes from Roy Porter, 'All Madness for Writing: John Clare and the Asylum', Hugh Haughton et al. (eds.), *John Clare in Context* (Cambridge: Cambridge University Press, 1994), pp. 259–78, p. 264. I review this important collection of essays in 'The John Clare Revival', *Literature and History*, 5 (1996), pp. 68–72. This is a review article which also contains commentary on John Lucas, *John Clare* (Plymouth: Northcote House, 1994). Porter's various studies of madness, for instance, *A Social History of Madness: Stories of the Insane* (London: Weidenfeld and Nicolson, 1987), which includes material on Clare (pp. 76–81), have influenced my approach.
2. As quoted in Anne Digby, *Madness, Morality and Medicine: A Study of the York Retreat, 1796–1914* (Cambridge: Cambridge University Press, 1985), p. 267. She reproduces the whole of Samuel W.'s case-notes as part of an appendix (pp. 262–78). It will be clear from the number of times that I cite her work that I am indebted to it. It still has to be said, however, that she (rather as Taylor sometimes did with Clare's poetry) tidies up Jepson's original notes when transcribing them: spelling is corrected, punctuation added and abbreviations filled out. This makes Jepson's text more authoritative and secure than it is in the original. There are also some transcription errors, as for instance when a reference to Samuel W.'s obscene remarks is omitted. To be fair, the manuscript, Borthwick Institute of Historical Research (BIHR), K/2/2, is often difficult to decipher. Digby's own text nevertheless shows that she endorses the favourable view of Jepson to be found in the propaganda for the Retreat. As will become clear, I take a more sceptical view.
3. BIHR, Retreat Casebook 1798–1828, K/2/1a, patient no. 85, p. 87. For the entries on his sisters, patients no. 67 and no. 110, see pp. 69 and 111. I am reluctantly following the convention of not providing most asylum inmates with their full names, which was presumably established to protect their families from the stigma of insanity, even though I think that this practice helps to infantilise them.
4. For an interesting piece of detective work on Sarah Walker, see Charles Nicholl, 'A Being Full of Witching', *London Review of Books* (18 May 2000), pp. 15–18. See also Anne Haverty, *The Far Side of a Kiss* (London, Chatto & Windus, 2000), for a fictional account of the relationship from Sarah's point of view.

5. These distinctions are discussed in *The Statistics of the Retreat; Consisting of a Report and Tables Exhibiting the Experience of that Institution for the Insane; from its Establishment in 1796 to 1840* (York: J.L. Linney, 1841), pp. 17–22.
6. Elizabeth F. was one of the inmates who was thought to suffer from 'lustiveness', BIHR, K/2/1A, p. 44. Her treatment included being spun around in a swing.
7. On the increasing links that were made between intemperance and madness, see D.J. Mellett, *The Prerogative of Asylumdom: Social, Cultural and Administrative Aspects of the Institutional Treatment of the Insane in Nineteenth-Century Britain* (London: Garland Publishers, 1982), pp. 76–85. For the development of the concept of 'moral insanity', see Eric T. Carlson and Norman Dain, 'The Meaning of Moral Insanity', *Bulletin of the History of Medicine*, 36 (1962), pp. 130–40. For an example of moral definitions of insanity, see George Man Burrows, as quoted in Vieda Skultans (ed.), *Madness and Morals: Ideas of Insanity in the Nineteenth Century* (London: Routledge & Kegan Paul, 1975), p. 38.
8. As quoted in Arthur Foss and Kerith Trick, *St. Andrew's Hospital Northampton: The First 150 Years (1838–1988)* (Cambridge: Granta, 1989), p. 81.
9. St. Andrews Hospital Archive, Northampton, CL1, p. 4. CL4, p. 31 contains a further reference to his bad language. I am grateful to Simon Kövesi for providing me with a transcript and more generally for stimulating discussions about Clare.
10. House Surgeon's Journal, 1834–7, Lawn 2/1/3, Lincolnshire Archives. Some of the relevant entries are: 30 August 1835 (admitted); 14 and 15 September (attacked nurse); 10 October (another escape attempt); 7, 9 and 13 November (indecent conduct); 26 December (more indecent conduct). She was discharged on 15 April 1836. Further details about her stay are in the Patient Ledger, Lawn 1/6/1, p. 388. The Physician's Journal, Lawn 2/2/4, reproduces the same sequence of events sometimes in the same words but it does at least make a point of recording her strong desire to be allowed to go home, which the House Surgeon ignores. Elaine Showalter's *The Female Malady: Women, Madness, and English Culture 1830–1980* (London: Virago, 1987) remains a very important study. See also Helen Small, *Love's Madness: Medicine, the Novel and Female Insanity 1800–1865* (Oxford: Clarendon Press, 1996).
11. As quoted in Digby, *Madness, Morality and Medicine*, p. 262.
12. As quoted in Digby, *Madness, Morality and Madness*, p. 266.
13. Roy Porter (ed.), John Haslam, *Illustrations of Madness* (London: Routledge, 1988), p. xxxviii. One of the inmates of the Retreat, James P., believed that he was being continually watched by government spies as a result of his disagreements with the state church, BIHR, K/2/1a, p. 84. He committed suicide shortly after admission.
14. I deal with the spy system in this period in the second half of *English Literature in History 1780–1830: Pastoral and Politics*.
15. Porter (ed.), *Illustrations of Madness*, p. xxxviii.
16. As quoted in Digby, *Madness, Morality and Medicine*, p. 268.
17. As quoted in Digby, *Madness, Morality and Medicine*, p. 272. The seventh day is Sunday.
18. BIHR, Retreat Case-Book 1, 1796–1828, K/2/1a, p. 69.
19. BIHR, K/2/1a, p. 271.

20. I am quoting the sub-title of Jacqueline Pearson's *Women's Reading in Britain 1750–1835: A Dangerous Recreation* (Cambridge: Cambridge University Press, 1999).
21. *A Sketch of the Origin, Progress, and Present State of the Retreat, An Institution near York, for the Reception of Persons Afflicted with Disorders of the Mind, among the Society of Friends* (London: W. Alexander and Son, 1828), p. 30. Emphasis added.
22. Jane Aaron, *A Double Singleness: Gender and the Writings of Charles and Mary Lamb* (Oxford: Clarendon Press, 1991), p. 109.
23. EG 2250, fol 12, letter dated 8 July 1840.
24. Thomas Arnold and others developed ideas on something called 'Nostalgic Insanity', *Observations on the Nature, Kinds, Causes, and Prevention of Insanity* (London: Richard Phillips, 1806), 2, 1, pp. 207–19, but this was quite specifically not seen as being an English malady.
25. John Taylor, Literary Correspondence and Family Papers, Derbyshire Record Office, D 1561, 774/1, Bundles of Correspondence: John Clare: Northamptonshire Poet. The letter is to Taylor's sister Elizabeth. Domestic violence is one of the many topics that I have discussed with Bob Heyes, although for reasons of space I was not able to use one possible piece of additional evidence to which he drew my attention. I, like many others, have benefited from the generous way in which he shares his knowledge.
26. Simon Kövesi (ed.), *John Clare: Love Poems* (Bangkok: M&C Services, 1999), p. xii.
27. For an account of Clare's journey, see Robin Jarvis, *Romantic Writing and Pedestrianism* (Basingstoke: Macmillan, 1997), pp. 159–62. For Clare's habit of walking, and its effects on his poetry, see Anne D. Wallace, *Walking, Literature and English Culture: The Origins and the Uses of Peripatetic in the Nineteenth Century* (Oxford: Clarendon Press, 1993), pp. 102–16.
28. See EG 2249, fols 304–5, letter dated 2 November 1837.
29. EG 2249, fol 377, letter dated 13 June 1837.
30. Lucas, *John Clare*, p. 2.
31. BIHR, K/2/1a, p. 227. He had approached Southey for help in getting the poem published. Southey's wife, Edith, incidentally spent a few months in the Retreat in 1834/5, complete with a servant and maid. According to some accounts of his last years, the Laureate himself possibly ought to have been there as well.
32. BIHR, K/2/1a, p. 191. Some of Lloyd's poems were reviewed in the *London Magazine*, 3, pp. 406–13. As I do not discuss Clare's use of the sonnet form, readers may wish to know that there is a collection of the sonnets that he wrote between 1832 and 1837, Eric Robinson et al. (eds.), *Northborough Sonnets* (Manchester: Carcanet, 1995).
33. David Masson (ed.), *The Collected Writings of Thomas De Quincey* (Edinburgh: Adam and Charles Black, 1889), 12, 2, p. 398.
34. Thomas Clarkson, *A Portraiture of Quakerism, as Taken from a View of the Moral Education, Discipline, Peculiar Customs, Religious Principles, Political and Civil Oeconomy and Character of the Society of Friends* (London: Longman, 1806), 3, 1, p. 124.
35. Tuke's views as quoted in Charles Taylor (ed.), *Samuel Tuke: His Life, Work and Thought* (London: Headley Brothers, 1900), p. 57. For more details on the Library at the Retreat, see *The Statistics of the Retreat*, p. 56.

36. As quoted in Digby, *Madness, Morality and Medicine*, p. 92.
37. *Description of the Retreat, an Institution near York for Insane Persons of the Society of Friends Containing an Account of its Origins and Progress, the Modes of Treatment and a Statement of Cases* (York: W. Alexander, 1813), p. 183.
38. *Description of the Retreat*, pp. 181–2.
39. *Description of the Retreat*, pp. 182–4, for quotation and full text of poem.
40. As quoted in Digby, *Madness, Morality and Medicine*, p. 275.
41. As quoted in Digby, *Madness, Morality and Medicine*, p. 276.
42. Marchand (ed.), *Byron's Letters and Journals*, 3, p. 179.
43. Some critics persist in reading the novel in either Freudian or Jungian terms. Sally Shuttleworth, *Charlotte Brontë and Victorian Psychology* (Cambridge: Cambridge University Press, 1996), is good at reconstructing specifically Victorian psychological models.
44. I deal in more detail with these events in *Jane Austen and Representations of Regency England*, Ch. 3.
45. See Joel Peter Eigen, *Witnessing Insanity: Madness and Mad-Doctors in the English Court* (New Haven: Yale University Press, 1995) for more details.
46. *A Treatise on Madness* (London: J. Whiston ..., 1758), p. 68.
47. *Description of the Retreat*, p. xii.
48. Christopher Hibbert (ed.), Louis Simond, *An American in Regency England: The Journal of a Tour in 1810–11* (London: Robert Maxwell, 1968), p. 109. Simond suggests that Jepson's wife, Catherine, was the person who really ran the Retreat, p. 110. Another American, John Griscom, has also left an account of the Retreat.
49. *The Works of the Reverend Sydney Smith* (London: Longman et al., 1859), 3, 1, p. 494. Other favourable reviews of the *Description* include *The Philanthropist*, 3, 1813, pp. 326–38.
50. BIHR, Minutes from the First 'Subscribers' Meeting on 1 January 1796 until the Committee Held on 29 February 1808, A/3/1a, entry for 28.10.1803. For the change in his financial arrangements, BIHR, Admissions Register 1796–1843, J/1/1, patient no. 85.
51. I am quoting from the title of William Parry-Jones, *The Trade in Lunacy: A Study in Private Madhouses in England in the Eighteenth and Nineteenth Centuries* (London: Routledge & Kegan Paul, 1972).
52. Details from BIHR, Visitors' Book 1798–1822, D/3/1b.
53. As quoted in Digby, *Madness, Morality and Medicine*, p. 273.
54. As quoted in Digby, *Madness, Morality and Medicine*, p. 86. The manuscript reference is BIHR, L/3/2, Tuke to S.W. Nicholl, 12 July 1814.
55. Sade's dramas provided the framework for Peter Weiss's play *The Persecution and Assassination of Marat as Performed by the Inmates of the Asylum of Charenton under the Direction of the Marquis de Sade* (London: John Calder, 1965).
56. D.D. Davies (trans.), Phillipe Pinel, *A Treatise on Insanity*... (Sheffield: W. Todd, 1806), pp. 52 and 87. For a good account of Pinel's career, see Jan Goldstein, *Console and Classify: The French Psychiatric Profession in the Nineteenth Century* (Cambridge: Cambridge University Press, 1987), Ch. 3.
57. Andrew Scull, *The Most Solitary of Afflictions: Madness and Society in Britain 1700–1900* (New Haven: Yale University Press, 1993), p. 5. Amongst other things Scull is good on the way in which 'moral management' was gradually

taken over by medical men, pp. 204–32. His materialistic approach leads him to describe Victorian asylums as becoming 'warehouses of the unwanted', p. 370. Nowadays unsold books are sent back to the warehouse. In Clare's case it was the writer himself who was warehoused.

58. Richard Howard (trans.), Michel Foucault, *Madness and Civilization: A History of Insanity in the Age of Reason* (London: Tavistock Publications, 1971), p. 64. I also discuss Foucault in my *Christopher Marlowe*.
59. *Madness and Civilization*, p. 224.
60. EG 2250, fol 21, letter dated 18 November 1841.
61. As quoted in Digby, *Madness, Morality and Medicine*, p. 145.
62. *An Account of the Imprisonment and Sufferings of Robert Fuller, of Cambridge...* (Boston: Printed for the Author, 1833), p. 23. Fuller claims that the insane do not even have the same legal rights as witches had in previous periods, p. 28.
63. *History and Present State of Brislington House near Bristol An Asylum for the Cure & Reception of Insane Persons. Established by Edward Long Fox M.D. AD 1804 and now Conducted by Francis & Charles Fox MDD* (Bristol: Light and Ridler, 1836), pp. 5 and 7. Catherine Jepson trained here.
64. *A Narrative of the Treatment Experienced by a Gentleman, During a State of Mental Derangement; Designed to Explain the Causes and the Nature of Insanity, and to Expose the Injudicious Conduct Pursued Towards Many Unfortunate Sufferers under that Calamity* (London: Effingham Wilson, 1838), pp. 91 and 98.
65. *A Narrative*, pp. 135–6.
66. *A Narrative*, p. 207.
67. Digby, *Madness, Morality and Medicine*, p. 151.
68. Nancy Tomes, 'The Great Restraint Controversy: A Comparative Perspective on Anglo-American Psychiatry in the Nineteenth-Century', W.F. Bynum et al. (eds.), *The Anatomy of Madness: Essays in the History of Psychiatry* (London: Tavistock Publications, 1985), 3, 2, pp. 190–225, p. 197.
69. BIHR, Female Visitors' Book 1816–1839, D/2/1a, entry for 4.11.1834. The visitors commented several times on the need for better washing and drying facilities, and more occasionally on the fact that inmates appeared to be allowed to stay in bed for too long.
70. John Conolly, *The Construction and Government of Lunatic Asylums and Hospitals for the Insane* (London: John Churchill, 1847), p. 36.
71. Q/ALp/3/1, Essex County Record Office.
72. As quoted in Digby, *Madness, Medicine and Morality*, p. 271.
73. *Madness and Civilization*, p. 247.
74. Q/ALp/3/1, Essex County Record Office.
75. *Description*, p. 150.
76. Matthew Allen, *Essay on the Classification of the Insane* (London: John Taylor, n.d.), pp. 47–8. I am grateful to my colleague Roger Cooter for providing me with references about Allen's career, as well as for reading the chapter as a whole, despite his other pressing commitments. To avoid any potential misunderstanding I may need to make it clear that Allen trained at the York Asylum rather than at the Retreat.
77. For more details on Tennyson, see Ann C. Colley, *Tennyson and Madness* (Athens: University of Georgia Press, 1983). Allen appears to have had a reputation amongst literary people as Thomas Campbell's son was at High

Beach at the same time as Clare. For more details, see William Beattie (ed.), *Life and Letters of Thomas Campbell* (London: Edward Moxon, London, 1859), 3, 2, pp. 400–12.

78. For publication details see endnote 1.
79. '"No Place Like Home": Reconsidering Matthew Allen and his "Mild System" of Treatment', *John Clare Society Journal*, 13 (1994), pp. 41–57. This is a sensible, useful account that does not take Allen at his own evaluation of himself.
80. See, for example, the account of Allen in Edward Storey, *A Right to Song: The Life of John Clare* (London: Methuen, 1982), pp. 256–74.

5 A government prison where harmless people are trapped: Regency poets and Victorian asylums

1. Details from Winifred Gerin, *Branwell Brontë* (London: Thomas Nelson, 1961). Some later writers are more suspicious and sceptical about the documentation for this trip. See, for example, Juliet Barker, *The Brontës* (London: Phoenix 1997), pp. 226–47. She suggests, amongst other things, that Branwell's behaviour on his return is not consistent with the feelings of rejection that may have been caused by this London trip. Perhaps this was just another one of his stories. There is a short article on Branwell's alcoholism by John Kent in *Yorkshire Medicine*, 6, 1994, pp. 10–11. One of the pleasures of writing this book has been the opportunity to read or re-read some excellent literary biographies by Barker herself, Grevel Lindoop, my colleagues Richard Holmes (on P.B. Shelley and Coleridge) and Andrew Motion, and others. Jonathan Bate's forthcoming biography of Clare promises to maintain this very high standard. His *The Song of the Earth* (London: Picador, 2000) contains important work on Clare. The title of this section is taken from Chuck Palahniuk, *Fight Club* (London: Vintage, 1997), from which I have also borrowed a few other phrases. There is a film version.
2. Pierce Egan, *Boxiana; or Sketches of Ancient and Modern Pugilism...* (London: Sherwood et al., 1818), 2, p. 212. Many of the details in this section are taken from the four-volume edition of *Boxiana* (1812, 1818, 1821 and 1824). The fourth volume was probably not by Egan. There was a fifth volume in 1829. I discuss Egan in 'Pierce Egan and the Representation of London', R. Jarvis and P. Martin (eds.), *Reviewing Romanticism* (Basingstoke: Macmillan, 1992), pp. 154–69. J.C. Reid, *Bucks and Bruisers: Pierce Egan and Regency England* (London: Routledge & Kegan Paul, 1971) is an important study. John Ford, *Prizefighting: The Age of Regency Boximania* (Newton Abbot: David and Charles, 1971) remains one of the better social histories. More recent studies include Dennis Brailsford, *Bareknuckles: A Social History of Prizefighting* (Cambridge: Lutterworth Press, 1988). See also Tom Bates, 'John Clare and Boximania', *John Clare Society Journal*, 13 (1994), pp. 5–17. Louis Golding, *The Bare-Knuckle Breed* (London: Hutchinson & Co., 1952), is a novelistic historical account. There is no evidence that Clare read Hazlitt's famous essay which was published in *The New Monthly Magazine* rather than in the *London*. It seems likely though, given his generally favourable opinion of Hazlitt's writings and his own passion for boxing. For the American ring,

see Elliott J. Gorn, *The Manly Art: Bare-Knuckle Prize Fighting in America* (Ithaca: Cornell University Press, 1986). I discuss Edward Bond's play about Clare, *The Fool*, first performed at the Royal Court in 1975, which explores relationships between boxing and poetry, in my *Pastoral and Politics*.

3. Randall's Challenge is one of the texts include in Tim Chilcott's excellently conceived edition, *John Clare: The Living Year 1841* (Nottingham: Trent Editions, 1999), p. 143, which freezes the frame to show a writer at work across a year. Trent Editions, a new imprint which may not yet be widely known outside the UK, do an important job in recovering a range of neglected writings in well-produced volumes.
4. Marchand (ed.), *Byron's Letters and Journals*, 9, p. 12.
5. Marchand (ed.), *Byron's Letters and Journals*, 3, p. 216.
6. For more details, see Benita Eisler, *Byron: Child of Passion, Fool of Fame* (London: Hamish Hamilton, 1999), pp. 102–3, and Marchand (ed.), *Byron's Letters and Journals*, 1, p. 169. Paul Magriel (ed.), *The Memoirs of the Life of Daniel Mendoza* (London: B.T. Batsford, 1951), contains a print of Byron sparring with Jackson, p. 45. Pierce Egan's *Life in London* has an illustration of Jackson's rooms, opposite p. 254. The homosexuality of Byron and his circle, which may help to explain the appeal of Jackson to them, is discussed in Louis Crompton, *Byron and Greek Love: Homophobia in 19th-Century England* (London: Faber and Faber, 1985). I discuss aspects of Byron's sexuality in 'The Loathsome Lord and the Disdainful Dame: Byron, Cartland and the Regency Romance', Frances Wilson (ed.), *Byromania: Portraits of the Artist in Nineteenth- and Twentieth-Century Culture* (Basingstoke: Macmillan, 1999), pp. 166–83.
7. *Boxiana*... (London: Sherwood, 1812), 1, p. 287.
8. Marchand (ed.), *Byron's Letters and Journals*, 3, p. 221.
9. Joyce Carol Oates, *On Boxing* (London: Bloomsbury, 1987), p. 30. Norman Mailer's *The Fight* (London: Penguin, 1991; 1st pub. 1975) touches very briefly on this aspect of boxing when it suggests that a 'man gets into the ring to attract admiration', p. 49. Mailer is attracted towards boxers because he identifies with them. Other writers, for instance George Bernard Shaw, were more conscious of differences.
10. For Cobbett's views, see John Derry (ed.), *Cobbett's England: A Selection from the Writings of William Cobbett* (London: Parkgate Books, 1997), pp. 172–80. This belief that Englishness was intimately bound up with a preference for fists over other weapons occurs again and again later on in popular fiction (e.g. Sherlock Holmes, Bulldog Drummond, Raffles). Cobbett blamed the Jews for corrupting pugilism. Later accounts such as Borrow's *Lavengro: The Scholar, The Gypsey, The Priest* (1851) stressed the way in which Spring and others represented the yeoman values of old England. A government spy slipped into a boxing club in Lobster Lane, Norwich to see whether the secretive Fancy might provide a front for political subversion, but found that this was not the case, Public Record Office, H0/40/13, fol 29.
11. 'John Clare's London Journal: A Peasant Poet Encounters the Metropolis', *Wordsworth Circle*, 23 (1992), pp. 172–5, p. 174. This is a very good short account of Clare's changing and ambivalent attitudes towards London. It implies, however, that Clare was watching prize-fighting proper rather than watching sparring with gloves, whereas there is no evidence that he ever

attended bareknuckle (and he would not have been able to do this in central London anyway). This is not being pedantic as it adds another level to the wish-fulfilment side of his relationship with boxing.

12. For more details about *Memoirs* and its reception, see Angela Thirkell, *The Fortunes of Harriette: The Surprising Career of Harriette Wilson* (London: Hamish Hamilton, 1936). Frances Wilson is currently writing what promises to be an exciting new biography.
13. For a discussion of this film see Peter Cochran, 'The Life of Byron, or Southey was Right?', and Ramona M. Ralston and Sidney L. Sondergard, 'Screening Byron: The Idiosyncrasies of the Film Myth', Wilson (ed.), *Byromania*, pp. 66–8 and 141–3. Although I agree that this was meant to be an unflattering representation of Byron, I still feel that Richard Chamberlain's reputation, presence and performance undercuts this at times.
14. This doodling by Clare is reprinted in Chilcott (ed.), *John Clare: The Living Year 1841*, p. 142. 'The Separation' is reproduced in Bernard Grebanier, *The Uninhibited Byron: An Account of his Sexual Confusion* (London: Peter Owen, 1971), p. 294. The wordplay is quite complicated: Biron was the archaic way of spelling Byron's name, and the Duke of Wellington was of course known as the Iron Duke.
15. J.W. and Anne Tibble (eds.), *The Prose of John Clare*, p. 224.
16. See Janet Todd, *In Adam's Garden: A Study of John Clare's Pre-Asylum Poetry* (Gainesville: University of Florida Press, 1973), for the work that is being done by terms like ape and aping in Clare's satirical writings, pp. 61–2.
17. Gilchrist sketches in some of the background to this controversy in letters to Clare. See EG 2245, fol 237 and fol 243, letters dated 24 and 26 November 1820. The controversy was discussed in the *London Magazine*, 3, pp. 593–607. Gilchrist (as will be seen) was one of the people who gave Clare copies of Byron's poetry. Eliza Emmerson, perhaps surprisingly given the way in which she appeared to line up so squarely behind Radstock and his crusade against vice, was also a great fan of Byron's work. Ever affectionate, she declared that '*two* poets only have my affections. Ld Byron and yourself', EG 2246, fol 114, letter dated 30 September 1822. Clare left her his copies of Byron in his will.
18. As quoted in J.W. and Anne Tibble (eds.) *The Prose of John Clare*, pp. 206–10.
19. Tannahill was a Scottish weaver who drowned himself in 1810 after failing to find a publisher for a second volume of poetry. Stephen Duck, an agricultural labourer whose career had established many of the archetypes in the script for peasant-poets, had drowned himself back in 1756.
20. For John Scott's profile of Byron, see *London Magazine*, 3, pp. 50–61.
21. For more details, see Haslett, *Byron's Don Juan and the Don Juan Legend*, pp. 36–66. It is not known whether Clare attended performances of *Don Juan*. All that can be said is that in the years of his first three visits to London (1820, 1822 and 1824) the figure of Juan was enjoying a popularity that went beyond Byron's poem. This may have been an additional reason for Clare to write his 'Don Juan' in the asylum. As mentioned, time and again he returns to the earlier 1820s when it still seemed possible for him to realise his great expectations. Austen went to a stage version of the Don Juan story at the Lyceum in 1816 and was not amused. Egan's lads attend a performance of *Don Giovanni* in *Life in London*. The popularity of

'underworld' dramas allowed the *London Magazine* to offer an amusing parody of them, 5, pp. 436–43, probably by Reynolds.

22. Camille Paglia, *Sexual Personae: Art and Decadence from Nefertiti to Emily Dickinson* (London: Penguin, 1991), p. 352. I mentioned in passing in the first chapter that Byron's popularity was like that of some of today's rock and pop stars. Paglia reads his career alongside that of Elvis Presley.
23. Wilson (ed.), *Byromania*, p. 1.
24. Although it is conventional to distance Austen and Byron like this, some Byron critics suggest interesting points of similarity, for instance between Aurora Raby in *Don Juan* and Fanny Price in *Mansfield Park* (1814). I have also argued more generally in *Jane Austen and Representations of Regency England* that the Regency novels (one of which was published by John Murray, Byron's publisher) remain fascinated by Byronic males even in the act of rejecting them.
25. See James Soderholm, *Fantasy, Forgery and the Byron Legend* (Lexington: University Press of Kentucky, 1996), which has some particularly original things to say about Byron's relationship with Caroline Lamb. Like Soderholm, Nicola J. Watson in *Revolution and the Form of the British Novel 1790–1825: Intercepted Letters, Interrupted Seductions* (Oxford: Clarendon Press, 1994) is fascinated by Lamb's forgery of a letter from Byron giving her permission to take a miniature portrait from his publishers during her wider analysis of the part played by the sentimental letter in this relationship, pp. 176–92. If Byron's *Don Juan* is his reply to *Glenavron*, perhaps Clare's 'Don Juan' is his reply to Patty Clare for the way in which she may colluded, or seemed to collude, in his imprisonment.
26. This reading is developed by Peter W. Graham, *Don Juan and Regency England* (Charlottesville: University Press of Virginia, 1990), which is a good study.
27. Philip W. Martin, *Byron: A Poet Before His Public* (Cambridge: Cambridge University Press, 1982), p. 187. In a later, more explicitly theoretical piece, Martin modifies to some extent his earlier position by insisting on the carnivalesque, dialogic nature of the poem, 'Reading *Don Juan* with Bahktin', Nigel Wood (ed.), *Don Juan* (Buckingham: Open University Press, 1993), pp. 90–121.
28. Details from Haslett, *Byron's Don Juan and the Don Juan Legend*, p. 150.
29. Anne Barton, 'John Clare Reads Lord Byron', *Romanticism*, 2 (1996), pp. 127–48. This is one of the best pieces of recent Clare criticism, to which I am much indebted. See also Philip W. Martin, 'Authorial Identity and the Critical Act: John Clare and Lord Byron', John Beer (ed.), *Questioning Romanticism* (Baltimore: Johns Hopkins University Press, 1995), pp. 71–91, and Edward Strickland, 'Boxer Byron: A Clare Obsession', *Byron Journal*, 17 (1989), pp. 57–81. For a good introduction to Byron's poem, see Barton, *Byron: Don Juan* (Cambridge: Cambridge University Press, 1992) in the Landmarks of World Literature series. She follows others such as Cecil Y. Lang by suggesting that a character who is eventually named as John Johnson might have been based on Gentleman Jackson.
30. For more details, see Andrew Elfenbein, *Byron and the Victorians* (Cambridge: Cambridge University Press, 1995). Carlyle's relationship with Byron, discussed in Chapter 3 here, is more complicated than I have been able to

show. There is also a fascinating Afterword looking at the way in which Anne Lister, a Regency lesbian, is able to appropriate Byron for her own relationships. Clare's boxer Byron was not the only Byron that was available.

31. As quoted in George Paston and Peter Quennell (eds.), *To Lord Byron: Feminine Profiles Based Upon Unpublished Letters 1807–1824* (London: John Murray, 1939), p. 159. Byron sends her some money. Another of the 'scandalous Regency ladies' of the 1820s, Madame Vestris, whose lovers were known as the Vestreymen, had sung a version of Clare's 'In Infancy' in 1820, although he had not be able to attend the performance. For her reputation see William W. Appleton, *Madame Vestris and the London Stage* (New York: Columbia University Press, 1974), pp. 17–48. As indicated, many Victorians were keen to distance themselves from such figures.
32. *Byron's Don Juan and the Don Juan Legend*, p. 130.
33. Elaine Feinstein (ed.), *John Clare: Selected Poems* (London: University Tutorial Press, 1968), p. 7. The view is endorsed by Eric Robinson and dissented from by John Barrell. Feinstein is yet another writer who has been involved in promoting Clare, the writer's writer.
34. See EG 2249, fols 304–5, letter from Henry Clay dated 29 October 1835.
35. Lynne Pearce, 'John Clare's *Child Harold*: The Road Not Taken', Susan Sellers (ed.), *Feminist Criticism: Theory and Practice* (London: Harvester Wheatsheaf, 1991), pp. 143–56. She also discusses 'Child Harold' in 'John Clare's Child Harold: A Polyphonic Reading', *Criticism*, 39 (1989), pp. 139–57. There are no facsimile editions of the notebooks that I know of, despite the insistent and persistent claims that we are being offered something called authentic Clare.
36. Although, as indicated, Egan was an important influence on Clare (which has not been fully recognised), there were a number of other guides to 'flash'. See, for example, Noel McLachlan (ed.), *The Memoirs of James Hardy Vaux Including His Vocabularly of the Flash Language* (London: Heinemann, 1964). This was first published in 1819 and was enthusiastically reviewed in the *London Magazine*. See K.C. Phillipps, *The Language of Thackeray* (London: Andre Deutsch, 1978), Ch. 2, 'Regency English in the Victorian Period', for an account of the way in which Regency slang becomes archaic in the earlier Victorian period.
37. George MacLennan, *Lucid Interval: Subjective Writing and Madness in History* (Leicester: Leicester University Press, 1992), p. 135.
38. Edward Mendelson (ed.), *The English Auden: Poems, Essays and Dramatic Writings 1927–1939* (London: Faber and Faber, 1977), p. 172.
39. Queen Victoria was not particularly popular at the beginning of her reign as a result of her dependence on Lord Melbourne and events such as the Bedchamber Scandal. See Robert Bernard Martin, *Enter Rumour: Four Early Victorian Scandals* (London: Faber and Faber, 1962), Ch. 1. Melbourne was Lady Caroline Lamb's husband.
40. Blunden's essay, 'John Clare: Beginner's Luck', is reprinted in *John Clare Society Journal*, 15 (1996), pp. 5–10. See also *John Clare: Poems Chiefly from Manuscript* (London: Richard Cobden-Sanderson, 1920).

Further Reading

Although by no means at all comprehensive, the endnotes still reference and comment on a reasonably wide range of books and essays about Clare himself (as well as ones on Regency and early Victorian cultural history more generally). They, together with the commentaries in the text of the argument itself, provide readers with opportunities to follow up the points made here.

The John Clare Society has produced a comprehensive guide to publications on Clare since 1970. This may be found on the John Clare web-site: http://human.ntu.ac.uk/clare. *The John Clare Society Journal*, 18 (1999), has a useful checklist of publications from 1993 to 1998, pp. 88–94. *The Journal*, 19 (2000) adds new material and brings the list up-to-date. These lists include academic dissertations which are not referenced in the notes here. Recent ones listed include important work such as Bob Heyes's study of provincial culture and Simon Kövesi's analysis of the later poetry. Part of Kövesi's project is to explore the complexity of Clare's representations of sexual identities in ways not attempted here. For an example of this work, see his essay on secrecy and femininity in *The John Clare Society Journal*, 18 (1999), pp. 51–63. The John Clare Society also produces a *Newsletter*.

When I have had the information, I have sometimes given details of work in progress. I understand that Jonathan Bate intends to complete his biography of Clare by the end of 2001. This will be a great help: there are still some silences in this story. The individual lives of agricultural labourers, even highly literate ones likes Clare, necessarily have moments of obscurity. Matters are also made worse in this case by the fact that the lives of alleged lunatics from whatever social background were shrouded in some secrecy. We know a certain amount about Clare's life sentence in the asylums: primarily from his own writings, as well as from the reports of others such as visitors, medical men and house-stewards. His experiences are in fact much better documented than those of most others, and yet there are still important gaps. I concentrated on Clare's earlier years as a published writer in the 1820s and then on the earlier asylum years. Readers will clearly need to consult other sources if working on other periods from this very long and productive literary life.

As Bate's biography will undoubtedly prove, our knowledge of Clare is increasing all the time: biographically, but also critically, editorially and historically. To take just one very quick example, I understand that this biography has important new material on the lives of Clare's family while he was in the asylums. My own very tentative suggestion (based on a remark by Taylor) that domestic violence might have played a part in the committals may well be proved to be wrong. The gaps and silences mean, certainly at the moment, that there have to be elements of speculation.

Because the web-site is so good and so up-to-date, I do not feel the need to add to it in any substantial way here. As mentioned in my Textual Note, there is a much more detailed chronology than I offer here on it by John Goodridge. In addition to references to related sites, this one includes some recent articles about Clare, a critical bibliography and a very useful first-line index to both published and unpublished poetry. Students at East Anglia who have used it regard it as one of the very best literary sites available (and I agree with them). It also contains details about the John Clare Society, which everyone who is working on Clare needs to contact. Students have also found the descriptive bibliography compiled by Goodridge for his edition of *The Independent Spirit: John Clare and the Self-Taught Tradition* a useful starting point. There are many bibliographical guides to the literature of the Romantic Period. The one edited by Michael O'Neill for the Clarendon Press in 1998 contains useful material on Clare by P.M.S. Dawson.

The John Clare Society Journal provides the best way of keeping in touch with the most recent developments. As academic books are usually completed at least a year before they are published, the current number of the *Journal,* 20 (2001) reminds me of some reading that I need to catch up on: James McKusick's *Green Writing: Romanticism and Ecology* and Goodridge and Kövesi's edition of essays, *John Clare: New Approaches*. I do not reference a recent biography that is reviewed in this number: Arnold Clay's *'Itching After Rhyme': A Life of John Clare.* As mentioned, I was not able to take advantage of the publication of *John Clare A Champion for the Poor: Political Verse and Prose,* but am now in a position to recommend it to readers.

Although I am very enthusiastic indeed about what I described in a recent review article as a revival of interest in Clare studies, I hope that I have also still given a sense of the importance of some of the earlier critical work. One of the things that I was reminded of in writing this book was the quality of some of the work by, amongst others, Barrell, Chilcott, Storey, Todd and the Williamses. Some, but alas not all, of them are still writing on Clare. I was also reminded of the way in which Johanne Clare's 1987 monograph posed some of the important historical questions.

I should perhaps make it clear that, although I have occasionally taken quotations from an edition called *Autobiographical Writings*..., Clare's editors, as I understand them, would recommend students to make exclusive use of a later edition called *John Clare by Himself,* published in 1996. This is described as extending, correcting and revising this earlier one (see my Textual Note for full publication details).

Although difficult to generalise given the activity around Clare, it seems to me that there may be two distinct and discernible trends in recent criticism, which are by no means competing ones. One is to continue to interrogate historically and critically some of the labels that were used (and are still sometimes used more subtly) to deny Clare's importance as a writer, to keep him in those 'leading strings'. The other has also been to assert his importance as a writer through close readings of his texts which relate him primarily to a wide range of other writers. I acknowledge the importance of this detailed textual work, while admitting that readers will need to go elsewhere for examples of it.

The full collection of letters addressed to Clare is available on microfilm from the British Library. My references to them just give a folio number and, when available, a date. I do not indicate, as more specialist publications might do, whether quotations come from the facing or reverse side of the folio, but I think that readers of a more general book like this still have enough information to follow them up if interested.

Perhaps, connecting Clare's long literary life with complicated mainstream cultural developments (Regency into Victorian) in a relatively short space, I may have sometimes made him sound like a difficult proposition for readers in the sense that he requires a lot of contextual knowledge (and there are many other equally important contexts such as forms of popular and culture not dealt with here). Contexts are important, but they are designed to make the lives and work of writers more accessible and knowable. Clare is a very exciting writer, as demonstrated by the current interest in him: of poetry obviously, but also of prose and letters (try, for example, his prose account of his escape from High Beach, *BH*, pp. 257–65).

Index

Page numbers given in *italics* refer to main entries. Material from the Acknowledgements, Chronology and Notes has not been systematically indexed, although I sometimes include some references from the Notes (usually in relation to Clare himself) to allow readers to follow up particular topics. In most cases a single reference in the argument not directly related to Clare has not merited inclusion in the Index. I have not indexed the Further Reading section. Shortened titles have sometimes been used for Clare's works.